# MEDICINES THAT KILL

*The Truth a[...]*
*Hidden Epidemic*

## JAMES L. MARCUM, MD

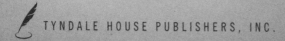

TYNDALE HOUSE PUBLISHERS, INC.

Visit Tyndale online at www.tyndale.com.

Visit Dr. Marcum's website at www.heartwiseministries.org.

*TYNDALE* and Tyndale's quill logo are registered trademarks of Tyndale House Publishers, Inc.

*Medicines That Kill: The Truth about the Hidden Epidemic*

Designed by Erik M. Peterson

Edited by Susan Taylor

The patient accounts in this book are real. The patients' names have been changed to protect confidentiality.

ISBN 978-1-4143-6885-6

Printed in the United States of America

| 19 | 18 | 17 | 16 | 15 | 14 | 13 |
|----|----|----|----|----|----|----|
| 7  | 6  | 5  | 4  | 3  | 2  | 1  |

*This book is dedicated to my patients—past, present, and future—who have been my inspiration. Your prayers, encouragement, and love have made you a part of this book.*

# Contents

# Acknowledgments

This book would never have been possible without a loving God Who gave me the strength, talent, and courage to convey new ideas. I hope this work is pleasing in Your sight.

A special note of gratitude to my loving wife, Sonya, and my children, Kelli and Jake, who had to share my time as this project moved forward.

Charles Mills provided important ideas and helped so much in the formulation of this book. Charles, you are a kindred spirit.

I also want to acknowledge Michael Bell, a partner in ministry and on the Heartwise Ministry team, who takes these ideas to the world via radio, television, and the Internet. I deeply appreciate your work and dedication.

I want to thank my family at Tyndale. Susan Taylor carefully edited the book while providing valuable input to improve the manuscript. You are a joy to work with. John Farrar, your ideas and faith in this book made the entire process a growing experience for me. April and Kristy, your work in getting this book to reach the world is priceless.

Last, I thank all my friends and family who have been praying and supporting this book. This book is a message, and I happen to be the messenger. To everyone else involved in any way and to a loving God, I say thank you.

# Disclaimer

This book is not meant to be a substitute for medical advice, diagnosis, and treatment by a trained medical professional. Always consult with your physician about your medical conditions and before altering your medications or your health routine.

# PART 1

# THE PROBLEM

*My people are destroyed from lack of knowledge.*
**HOSEA 4:6, NIV**

I FIRST MET DANA in the intensive care unit after she had undergone surgery to repair a damaged heart valve. The surgery was complicated by pulmonary hypertension, a condition in which the pressure in the pulmonary vessels (those in the lungs) is much higher than normal. This contributed to her abnormal heart rhythm and right-sided heart failure. Week after week this forty-five-year-old in the prime of life became weaker and weaker, and the specialists, the medications, the ventilator, the feeding tube, the dialysis, and everything else modern medicine had to offer could not "fix" the problems.

Before her illness, Dana had not smoked, drunk, or used

illicit drugs. She had been a member of the track team in high school. In fact, years before, an episode of palpitations had resulted in a thorough medical evaluation. This included blood work, a complete history and physical, an electrocardiogram, a twenty-four-hour monitor, and an echocardiogram. Everything was normal. Dana's palpitations turned out to be from drinking too much caffeine and vanished when Dana decreased her caffeine intake and drank more water.

Dana was happily married with two children. Her daughter, Rhonda, was engaged to be married and was graduating from college the same month as her wedding. As one might expect, Dana and her daughter were excited about the upcoming event, and Dana was involved in all the details.

In preparation for the wedding, Dana wanted to lose some weight. She saw her family doctor, who recommended a diet and a moderate exercise program. But Dana wanted a quick fix. With the upcoming wedding, she felt she did not have the time to lose the weight slowly as her doctor suggested. Some friends had lost weight quickly with a diet medication called Fen-Phen. Dana got a prescription for the medication and lost twenty pounds quickly.

At first she felt great, with boundless energy. She was proud when others noticed her girlish figure returning and commented on how good she looked. However, this energetic feeling was only temporary. After a while, even the simplest activity left Dana short of breath, and she was tired all the time. Something was terribly wrong. She saw her doctor, who discovered a heart valve problem. How could this have happened? She had never had a heart problem before.

It was about this time that the Mayo Clinic first reported twenty-four cases of heart valve damage attributed to Fen-Phen. Yes, the medication had damaged Dana's heart valve to the point that nothing more could be done to help her. She passed away soon after her daughter's wedding and graduation.

Let me ask you a question: What do Michael Jackson, Whitney Houston, Heath Ledger, John Belushi, Chris Farley, Anna Nicole Smith, Elvis Presley, and yes, Dr. Sigmund Freud have in common? No, it is not that they are entertainment icons or psychoanalysts. Their deaths were the results of the use of various medications—yes, medications. Did these people die because of a lack of knowledge? Perhaps. But these are just a few of the well-known persons whose deaths have made front-page headlines. Let me tell you, we have a rapidly escalating problem. I do not want one more person to die from a lack of knowledge. Medications can kill. Medications do kill. Medications have killed. Medications are killing, and not nearly enough is being said. I hope to change this.

As I sat down to write the most significant introduction in my life as a physician, I found myself wondering, *What can I write to touch your heart? What can I write to help you to grasp the enormity of the problem? What words can I use that will enter your mind and change the way you think and live?* In just a few short pages these words have the opportunity to save more lives than anything else I have done in my profession as a cardiologist. Words are sometimes inadequate when faced with a cultural and worldwide problem. Words seem just as inadequate when I want to shake up the status quo, open your eyes, and help you to know the truth.

If doctors had known, most of them would not have written three to four million prescriptions for Fen-Phen. William Osler, a highly respected Canadian physician and one of the founders of the medical school at Johns Hopkins Hospital, once said, "The person who takes medicine must recover twice, once from the disease and once from the medicine." With billions of prescriptions being written each year, medications are killing more and more individuals. I want to raise the possibility and make the case that medications are the leading cause of death, at least in North America, and perhaps in the world.

In 2010, according to the National Vital Statistics Report released in January 2012, cardiovascular disease was the number one cause of death, claiming 595,000 lives in that year. Cancer was the second leading cause of death, claiming 574,000 lives. Respiratory illnesses took 138,000 lives. These trends hold true throughout the world. The report also indicated that the incidence of deaths from cardiovascular causes was trending downward slightly and that cancer-related deaths were trending upward. Nowhere did the report mention that medications were a leading cause of death. But it should have.

One does not have to be a scientist to realize that there are hundreds of thousands of deaths never reported: deaths because of mistakes made during production of medications, including manufacturing and even labeling; and mistakes made by medical personnel, including doctors, nurses, and pharmacists. There are deaths that result from adverse reactions, including anaphylaxis (hypersensitivity); deaths to the unborn caused by medications taken by their mothers; deaths from overdoses and addictions, which are now at epidemic proportions; deaths from impairment caused by certain medications; and deaths from misuse and inappropriate use of medication, which are considerable. All these deaths must be added to the total number of deaths indicated by the government report. If we were able to factor these in, we would see that medications are the number one cause of death, far surpassing cardiovascular disease. Do I have an exact number? No. Do I have hard data? Yes and no. Do I have logic and a good deal of professional experience to back my claim? Keep reading.

It only makes sense that as more and more medications are prescribed and as more and more over-the-counter (OTC) drugs used for a myriad of symptoms find their way into our medicine cabinets, these numbers will continue to rise. I can say, with logic and with limited statistics, that death by medications is the number one cause of death, and the number continues to rise.

I am a physician trained in internal medicine and cardiology. I try to prevent deaths from cardiovascular disease. But it is plausible to conclude—after studying these numbers and thinking about the problem of medications—that my time seeing patients might be better spent combating deaths from medications and educating the world about the dangers of taking prescription and nonprescription medications. In the long run, I might save more lives!

We continue to read and hear about deaths due to terrorism, accidents, natural disasters, cardiovascular disease, cancer, and you name it. The time is now to hear about the deaths occurring every day at staggering rates from medications. Your friends, family members, neighbors, and citizens of the world are dying. Someone needs to speak out. Something needs to be done.

# 1

# MY MEDICAL HISTORY

*The doctor of the future will give no medicine,*
*but will interest his patient in the care of the human frame,*
*in diet and in the cause and prevention of disease.*
**—THOMAS EDISON**

"I'M GOING TO TEACH you about poison," the professor announced to my pharmacology class in medical school. At first I thought he was kidding. He wasn't.

I grew up in a medical family. My father was an anesthetist, and my mother a registered nurse. I remember hearing stories about happenings at work, both good and bad. Many of those stories involved medications. I remember a gentleman with lymphoma who received too much chemotherapy and died suddenly. There were occasional stories of adverse drug reactions. At an early age I was aware of the risks involved with medications.

As I went through medical school at the University of

Texas, I was inundated with material. Classes on the mechanism of medicines and how each affected the body fascinated me. We spent hour after hour studying pharmacology and learning when to use certain medications, the dangers involved, and the hoped-for chemical benefits.

When my residency in internal medicine began at the Medical Center of Delaware, it was my turn to practice—for the first time—what I'd learned in medical school. I well remember the first time I wrote orders for a patient in the hospital. I went over and over the order for a blood thinner called heparin, making sure it was perfect. I can still recall handing out my first prescription. The seriousness of those pen strokes hit me with full force. I was about to change someone's chemistry. In doing so, I could help sustain him, or I could kill him. That responsibility weighed heavily on my mind. I can remember so vividly the time I spent on the hematology (the study of blood)/oncology (the study of cancer) rotation, where I watched the effects of powerful chemotherapy drugs that poisoned the bone marrow, killing good cells as well as the bad cells. I remember all the transfusions needed to keep the red blood cells and platelets at adequate levels in these patients. When the white blood cells, the fighter cells, were wiped out, powerful antibiotics and antiviral and antifungal medications were prescribed to prevent infection. The patients were so weak and prone to many problems. I often thought, *Which is worse: the treatment or the disease?* The more I learned, the less I knew.

During my fellowship in cardiovascular disease at the

University of Kentucky, I witnessed firsthand the potency and potential of medications. Back then, as a heart-attack treatment we administered medicines called thrombolytics. These were very powerful blood thinners that could do one of two things—or both: abort a heart attack or cause dangerous bleeding. It wasn't easy explaining to patients that the medicine I had just prescribed could save their hearts *and* could also increase the likelihood of fatal bleeding in their heads or elsewhere in their bodies.

On a good day, the medications worked. On a bad day, an adverse reaction carried an innocent man or woman in my care to the very edge of eternity. I'm thankful that there were more good days than bad, and I began to see the incredible benefits of drugs used in tightly controlled environments. I recognized that using medications required skill and communication at various levels. Any medication had the potential to kill if used in the wrong amount, used for an inappropriate medical condition, delivered in the wrong way, or given to a weakened metabolism. Likewise, a breakdown of the system at any level would have dire consequences.

The medicines I administered to correct cardiovascular rhythms worked as advertised, bringing irregular heart rhythms back in line. But every once in a while, a heart would stubbornly head in the exact opposite direction. Even when I exercised extreme care, there were no guarantees.

I soon realized that medicines and treatments fell into a category best described as "medical risk management." Those risks could quickly become compounded if someone—the patient or the caregiver—wasn't absolutely clear on what he or she was doing. And there were always questions lurking in the back of my mind: *Is there a genetic risk here? Will this medicine cause an anaphylactic (hypersensitivity) reaction from previous contact with it? Have I missed anything? What can I do to help my patients avoid these deadly risks? Are there safer ways to control body chemistry? What are the long-term effects on the body?* It would be years before I began to uncover some of the answers.

As I moved into private practice, I soon learned our world was very, very sick. The line of patients waiting outside my door was never ending. Because of the workload, I was forced to spend less and less time educating patients about the medications I was prescribing. I kept wondering, *Will this do more harm than good? Will this cause bleeding? Will patients experience a dangerous heart rhythm? Will they become dehydrated and suffer kidney malfunction, thus making the medication more potent than it should be? Will patients take their medicines correctly, or at all? Have I given them enough information to reduce their risks?*

Then there were the pharmaceutical representatives who came calling. I remember one medication for cholesterol that hit the market. It was touted as the greatest way on the planet to lower cholesterol. Sure enough, it did, but soon Baycol was yanked off the shelves because it caused dangerous muscle damage called myositis. None of the representatives from pharmaceutical companies who came calling suggested that these medicines were dangerous. No one sat across from me in a well-tailored suit or perfectly pressed dress and acknowl-edged that the medicines should be tested more thoroughly and had a very real chance of killing people in my care. Sure, the dangerous aspects were mentioned, but usually in small print or at the short end of a long and glowing presentation. These companies wanted to help society but, I discovered, they were also in the business of making money. They needed to sell product—lots of product—to stay afloat.

## Who Am I?

I soon began to question my own thinking: *Why haven't I heard more about the dangers? Who am I to buck the system? Who am I to lift my head above the herd and say that some-thing is wrong?* That pharmaceutical "system" thrived under the unspoken assumption that there are no profits in mak-ing people well. Healthy people don't take medications. However, if a medication could make a patient feel better and yet not "fix" the problem, the company selling it would have itself a gold mine. Of course, killing people isn't a good idea either. And that's where the drug companies kept trip-ping over themselves.

My colleagues and I were becoming busier and busier. Just making it through each day was a challenge. Who had time to question the medical culture that was evolving around us? More and more medications were being devel-oped by megacompanies each year. Fast-tracking was mak-ing it easier to bring medications to the market. The FDA had more and more work to do with less staffing to do it. There were more and more top-quality advertisements blasting from television screens, from magazine ads, and from the briefcases of smiling drug company reps. We physicians— along with our patients—were being told over and over and over again, "You have to utilize these medications. If you don't, you're way behind the curve. You are not a good doctor." Even my patients started saying, "Hey, Doc, I saw this medicine on TV, and I think it's exactly what I need. Write me up a prescription, and I'll be on my way." In other words, they wanted a quick fix and weren't so worried about the long-term consequences.

As the sheer volume of drugs, ads, and profits soared, and I mean soared, a little voice in the back of my mind kept whispering, *Something isn't right here. This does not make sense.*

Society was being told that pills are the answer, but my patients kept coming back with the same illnesses year after year. Not only that, I was seeing and hearing firsthand about more and more deaths occurring as a direct result of taking medications.

Finally I decided that my job as a cardiologist was not confined to simply keeping people alive. I had to teach them how to protect themselves from the well-marketed world and how to live so they would not have to come see me again. I determined to do more than prescribe a dangerous medication. I wanted to tell anyone who would listen how to survive medication free, if possible.

But first I had to pull back the curtain and reveal the

hidden dangers in the pills and potions that my patients consumed. These dangers needed to be shouted from the rooftops and not merely whispered about in the academic corridors. I felt compelled to say what most in my profession wanted to say. I had to remind all who would listen that in spite of what the media and other physicians may tell you, medicines can kill and are a leading cause of death.

## Transcendent Power

Something else was happening to me during those years. I was feeling a growing need for a power in my life that transcended what I'd learned in medical school, what I'd heard from a hundred church pulpits, and what I'd experienced trying to be a Christian in a society that seemed determined to disconnect from God altogether.

I was born and raised in a Christian home. I attended church, sang hymns, read my Bible, and prayed. But for some reason, I never connected those activities to the world of health. More to the point, I never connected those spiritual activities to the building and maintaining of health. Christianity was something I did, something I believed, not something I used to stay healthy.

All that changed when I began to see a convergence taking place, a coming together of two elements—biblical theology and science. As scientists gained the tools necessary to peer further and further into what makes life possible, I found that my faithful Bible began to make more sense. It was as if modern researchers were seeking for proof to verify what my Bible teaches. Study after study seemed to underline certain passages, bringing to light their ancient truths. The Bible was a source of medical truth. This merging of science and the Bible changed the way I regarded Scripture and launched me on a search for healing that continues to this day. I realized that for the first time in history, science wasn't refuting Bible truth; science was proving it!

Health wasn't just about eating the right foods and getting sufficient exercise. It wasn't just about pills versus plants or organic versus conventional. In my search for truth, I came to realize that health is a by-product of a love relationship with God. It begins with Him loving us and ends with us loving Him. Everything else—every choice we make, every habit we overcome, every thought we think—must be a direct result of that growing connection we enjoy with the one who created us. The further we move away from that connection, the sicker we become.

So, if I was going to serve my patients to the best of my ability, I was going to have to include spiritual principles and what I call "biblical technology" right along with science and medicine. This biblical technology could change the chemistry of our bodies. I was going to have to learn to prescribe what was proven to work best, not just what smiling pharmaceutical representatives pushed under my nose week after week.

Were there substitutes for modern medicine as it relates to chronic conditions? Could I, in good conscience, suggest those substitutes to my patients as a way of healing their maladies?

I determined that was exactly what I was going to do. But first I had to take a long, hard look at both modern medicine and biblical technology to discover where each is needed and how to merge them into a single healing ministry. The journey wouldn't be easy, but it would certainly be worth it! I determined to find a way to let my patients know that medications have a place in healing but can also do harm and, in some cases, kill. The following chapters describe what I've learned on that journey.

✛

## LEADING CAUSES OF REPORTED DEATHS IN AMERICA*

| | | |
|---|---|---|
| 1. | Heart disease | 632,000 |
| 2. | Cancer | 600,000 |
| 3. | Stroke | 177,000 |
| 4. | Respiratory failure | 125,000 |
| 5. | Accidents | 122,000 |
| 6. | Diabetes | 72,000 |
| 7. | Pneumonia/flu | 56,000 |
| 8. | Kidney failure | 45,000 |

*Kenneth D. Kochanek, MD, et al, "Deaths: Final Data for 2009," *National Vital Statistics Reports* 60, no. 3 (December 29, 2011), 5. Available at www.cdc.gov /nchs/data/nvsr/nvsr60/nvsr60_03.pdf. Accessed October 26, 2012.

✛

# 2

# IT COULD HAPPEN TO YOU

*It is a wise man's part rather to avoid sickness
than to wish for medicines.*
**—SIR THOMAS MORE**

HAVE YOU EVER SAID, "That couldn't happen to me"? I hear the comment often in my own family. In fact, I'd be willing to bet you've said or thought the same thing at some point. A few years ago, my beautiful wife was traveling extensively in her work as a health care consultant. At the beginning of the week she would fly to her destination and then return home at the end of the week. Of course, I was always there to pick her up. One particular week she was in El Paso, Texas. She was scheduled to fly home on Friday, and I was eagerly awaiting her return to Lexington, Kentucky. When my wife had to call to tell me she was in St. Louis, she realized it *could* happen to her. She had gotten on the wrong plane and ended up in the wrong city. Today this seems comical, but if I remember correctly, I was not too amused that night.

You may be thinking, *How could this happen? Who would get on the wrong plane?* I am sure if you had asked my wife, a seasoned traveler, if that would ever happen to her, she would have said, "That could never happen to me." But for whatever reason, it did happen to her.

A few years ago we were enjoying a family vacation in Arizona. We were amazed and awed at the Grand Canyon, Sedona, and the beauties of Arizona in the spring. We were driving back to our hotel one evening when Jake, my young son, announced that he had to go to the bathroom. As every father with kids understands, sometimes it's just not convenient to stop. Besides, if I stopped every time someone had to go to the bathroom, we would never get anywhere. Needless to say, this was not the first time we'd encountered the situation, and Jake was quite adept at taking care of this problem in a bottle, which he proceeded to do. Soon the sun had vanished, and the vast desert was filled with darkness. We were within twenty minutes of our hotel, and I was being attentive to the busy roads near Scottsdale when I became thirsty and reached for a water bottle in the console of the rental car. It didn't take my taste buds more than a few seconds to realize I was drinking from the wrong bottle. If you had asked me if I would ever drink urine, I would have said emphatically, "That could never happen to me!" Well it did happen to me, and yes, similar misfortunes could happen to you.

Think honestly for a moment: How many times have

things that you never thought possible happened to you or to your family? Getting the wrong tickets to a movie, receiving the wrong food at a restaurant, or going the wrong way on a road—yes, these can happen to you. They have happened to me.

In my medical practice I see a similar problem. No one thinks a deadly mistake related to medications could happen to him or her, but with billions of prescriptions being written each year, mistakes—even deadly mistakes—could happen to you. Sometimes we have no control. The statistics say these mistakes are occurring. News reports say they are occurring. Medicines are killing, and that could happen to you. Now, please don't misunderstand. I am *not* saying that modern medications don't have their place. I'm a physician, and the use of medications is often part of the treatment I give, especially for acute medical conditions. The point I want to make, however, is that there can be a real and present danger with the use of medications, and we all need to become aware and do everything we can to minimize the risk.

Where do these risks come from? Some of them are the result of mistakes made in the production, distribution, or even labeling of the medicines. Others are the result of human error on the part of pharmacists, doctors, nurses, and other providers. These mistakes are increasing as our world experiences more and more symptoms. Then there are patient errors, which are increasing dramatically as people age. It never quite surprises me, as I would expect, when I hear of yet another mistake made by a patient or a caregiver.

Misuse (use of certain medications for something other than intended) is causing major problems as well. If we add these factors to the risks inherent in the medications themselves, we have a problem more common than you would think, a problem that could happen to you or to your loved ones.

I am sure I have made mistakes with medications. Patients make mistakes. Pharmaceutical companies make mistakes. Hospitals make mistakes. This type of problem is hard to admit and even harder to measure. And although we know these kinds of mistakes are made, we also know that medications are needed for the treatment of disease. I realize that it is not popular to say that the medical profession, the pharmaceutical companies, and society as a whole have a problem. But until we acknowledge the problem, we have little hope of finding a solution.

Before we go further, let me tell you about some patients who thought certain medical mistakes could not happen to them.

## A Tough Pill to Swallow

The middle-aged man was experiencing chest pain, or angina, on exertion, so his doctor prescribed a nitroglycerin patch to help alleviate the symptom. The medicine in the patch would dilate the coronary arteries and allow freer blood flow.

After a few weeks, at a follow-up appointment, the doctor asked the patient whether his chest pain had improved.

"Not really," the man said.

"Did you use the patches?" the doctor queried.

"Well, I quit taking them after a week," his patient responded. "They made me violently sick to my stomach, and I was dizzy all the time. I thought I was dying."

"Strange," the doctor said, with some degree of concern. "I have never had that problem with the patches before. The side effect I hear about most often is a headache. Were you using them as prescribed?"

"Absolutely," the patient said firmly. "And not only did they make me sick, I was having a very hard time swallowing them."

The doctor sat stunned for a moment, then quickly explained to his patient that the patches were meant to be placed on the skin, not swallowed.

The now-enlightened patient was able to adjust how he used his prescription and eventually gained some benefit. He was lucky. Thousands of people each year make similar mistakes and die.

It seems almost impossible to comprehend, but emerging evidence indicates that the high-tech, powerful, Food and Drug Administration–approved pills and potions we carry home from the pharmacy in those little white bags are failing to heal us. They are not "fixing" the problem. With alarming regularity, they are doing just the opposite, for a variety of reasons.

The man who was swallowing the patches likely never thought that the medication his doctor prescribed to help him could have killed him. Fortunately it did not, but it could have happened to him. And it could happen to you.

## Knee Replacement

Martha, age seventy, had debilitating arthritis in both knees. The condition had progressed to the point that she could no longer walk without extreme pain. She had tried pain medication with little success. She thought the pain pills made her goofy. Her orthopedic surgeon recommended surgery to replace both knee joints. With the exception of her knees, Martha was healthy. She had no problems with her heart, lungs, or kidneys. Her internist thought the risk of surgery would be low. When the time came, the surgery went well from a technical perspective; however, Martha developed an infection in her lungs in the postoperative period. The cause was a bacteria known as methicillin-resistant staphylococcus aureus, or MRSA, which is resistant to many antibiotics.

Martha was started on an antibiotic combination of vancomycin, rifampin, and gentamicin to combat the infection. During that time, her medical team noted that her kidneys were being adversely affected by the antibiotics and that kidney function would need to be monitored closely. They also felt that Martha was not strong enough to go home and transferred her to a rehabilitation facility. The infection specialist left detailed recommendations for the dosing of the antibiotics, but these were lost in the transfer, and Martha's kidney function declined further. Eventually, her kidneys failed completely from the toxicity of the antibiotics, and she had to begin dialysis. But in Martha's weakened condition, her body just could not withstand the effects of the dialysis, and Martha died.

Modern medications can be lethal even when used as they are designed to be. In Martha's case, the antibiotics eliminated the infection; in the process, however, they damaged her kidneys. Medications can be toxic. They are often unforgiving of any misuse. Martha's medical team did not think this was possible, but it happened to them and to Martha. And it could happen to you.

## The Cascade Effect

Mr. Bell was admitted to the hospital for treatment of severe dehydration. He had undergone treatment for renal cell carcinoma, a cancer of the kidneys. The chemotherapy and radiation had left him unable to eat or drink, and the resulting lack of fluid intake had compromised Mr. Bell's kidney function. His doctor ordered intravenous fluids (normal saline) to replenish the volume of water in his body, but as he received the intravenous fluids, Mr. Bell became increasingly short of breath and his body became swollen. The nursing staff summoned the doctor, who prescribed a medicine to help remove the excess fluid. But Mr. Bell's condition continued to deteriorate. He also developed atrial fibrillation, an abnormal heart rhythm, which further compromised his health.

Family members, already worried, became even more concerned when one of them noticed that the intravenous fluids, which were flowing continuously, were labeled not saline but oxytocin. This medication, oxytocin, is sometimes given to pregnant women to induce labor. The medication was promptly discontinued and the medical team treated Mr. Bell for congestive heart failure. But because of the heart failure, his cancer treatment was discontinued.

Eventually Mr. Bell was discharged and given medications for heart failure. A few months later he returned to be evaluated by a cardiologist. Testing revealed that the abnormal rhythm had normalized and heart function was within the limits of normal. His cardiac medications were discontinued. The earlier symptoms had been caused by the continuous oxytocin drip. Sadly, by the time Mr. Bell made it back to the oncologist, his cancer had spread and eventually took his life. A single mistake initiated a cascade of adverse events. This happened to Mr. Bell, and it could happen to you.

## Asthma Attack

Emma was rushed to the hospital with yet another asthma attack. Her parents had been through the routine before. Childhood asthma attacks were no stranger to them, and they knew the drill. Emma received oxygen and intravenous medications. She and her family were traveling out of state, so her regular pediatrician was not available. The physician treating Emma ordered a medication to ease her labored breathing. Tragically, someone made a math mistake: the decimal point was in the wrong place, and Emma received the wrong dose. She suffered a seizure from which she was unable to recover.

Dosing mistakes are more common in children than in adults because the dosing varies, usually according to a patient's weight. Pediatric patients suffer up to an 11 percent rate of medical error, much higher than their adult counterparts, which one study found was approximately 6 percent.[1] Emma's parents did not think this could happen to them.

## Dangerous Rhythms

Cardiologists use medications to regulate abnormal heart rhythms every day. One rhythm I treat frequently is atrial fibrillation. As I looked through the risks of the medications used to treat this problem, I learned that all the medications have the potential to cause deadly rhythms if used inappropriately. They also have the potential to cause deadly rhythms even if used appropriately.

Sam was taking a medication called sotalol. The medication had worked well for a time, but gradually Sam was having more and more episodes of atrial fibrillation. His heart was going into this abnormal rhythm for several hours every day. His active lifestyle was being "messed up." He assumed, according to his family, that if he needed to, he could take an extra pill for these episodes. The "extra pill or two" triggered an abnormal rhythm called ventricular tachycardia. The paramedics who responded to the emergency call while Sam was on his beach vacation were unable to restore a stable rhythm, and he died.

Again, all medications for heart rhythms have the potential for lethal problems, even when used appropriately. Risks and benefits must be constantly assessed. Sometimes the risk of using a medication is greater than the risks associated with the symptoms being treated. We must realize that all medications have the potential to create problems, including death. One reason is that while a particular medicine is busy attacking a central ailment via a specific chemical pathway—often with satisfactory results—it can be working tirelessly in the background wreaking havoc with other delicate body systems and their supporting organs. And yes, it could happen to you.

—— + ——

### DR. MARCUM'S TOP TEN DANGEROUS CLASSES OF MEDICATIONS

**1. OPIOID PAINKILLERS.** These include medications sold under the names Lortab, Oxycontin, and Vicodin. They can depress respiration (breathing) and adversely affect many other medications. The immune system becomes compromised. The hormonal balances change. Dependence is a possibility.

**2. CHEMOTHERAPY.** These medications kill good cells as well as bad cells. The cells (white blood cells, red blood cells, and platelets) produced by the bone marrow are poisoned, making infections, anemia, and bleeding more likely. Chemotherapy can also damage organs such as the heart, liver, and kidneys.

**3. BLOOD THINNERS.** Thrombolytics and warfarin are very potent, and a little bleeding can become fatal, especially if it occurs in the head or is undiscovered for a time. All cells in the body need the oxygen the red blood cells carry.

**4. ANTIARRHYTHMICS.** Medications such as amiodarone, sotalol, dofetilide, mexiletine, and beta-blockers (sold under such names as Coreg, Tenormin, Lopressor) can help stabilize an abnormal heart rhythm but can also cause dangerous fast and slow rhythms. They must be used with extreme care.

**5. STEROIDS.** Medicines sold under such names as Solu-Medrol, hydrocortisone, and Decadron are a few of the steroids on the market. Over a long period of time these medications can contribute to fluid retention, diabetes, weakened immune systems and subsequent infections, osteoporosis, increased weight and its resultant problems, gastrointestinal bleeding, reopening of wounds (dehiscence), and adrenal problems.

**6. DIURETICS.** These medications remove fluid from the body. Drugs sold under such names as Lasix, Demedex, metolazone, hydrochlorothiazide, and Aldactone are a few of these that are frequently prescribed. These medications can change the balance of electrolytes (minerals that affect many of the metabolic processes in the body), which could cause lethal heart arrhythmias. They also can dehydrate the body and cause kidney and blood pressure problems. If kidney function is compromised, the concentration of many other medications in the body increases.

**7. NONSTEROIDAL ANTI-INFLAMMATORY DRUGS (NSAIDS).** These medications help decrease inflammation but may cause dangerous gastrointestinal bleeding or provoke heart attacks.

**8. ATTENTION DEFICIT DISORDER MEDICATIONS.** Drugs sold under the names Ritalin and Adderal can cause dangerous heart rhythms.

**9. DIABETES MEDICATIONS.** Insulin, glucophage, and the rest lower blood sugar. But a blood-sugar level that is too low is also very bad.

**10. ANTIDEPRESSANTS.** Some, such as Prozac and Zoloft, have been associated with a greater risk of suicide.

+

## Chemotherapy

I was asked to evaluate Larry because his heart was racing. He was in the intensive care unit and doing poorly. He had lymphoma, a cancer of the lymphatic system, which had spread, and he had received his second round of chemotherapy. The good thing is, chemotherapy kills the bad cells that are dividing inappropriately. The bad thing is, chemotherapy damages the good cells as well. In Larry's case the bone marrow had been damaged. The numbers of both Larry's white blood cells (needed to fight infections) and his hemoglobin and platelets (which aid in oxygen transport and clotting) were dangerously low. He had picked up an infection from an abrasion on his skin. Normally this would not be a medical emergency, but because of his compromised state, he was unable to fight the infection. The infection entered his bloodstream, and Larry developed multi-organ system failure from the toxins released by the unhindered bacteria. Larry's heart was doing everything it could do to help maintain a healthy blood pressure, but the infection was too strong. Larry was only forty-five.

## Research

There's also the matter of research. Because pharmaceutical companies invest millions of dollars to develop new medications, they need to put their products on the market quickly in order to recoup the money they've spent developing them. Unfortunately, we as a society are often unwittingly acting as guinea pigs. If you doubt that statement, consider this question: What are the long-term results of taking a cholesterol-lowering statin, the most prescribed medication in America? The truth is, we don't know. But we will find out soon enough, because the first generation of statin takers are beginning to age. If history is any guide, the more medicines we ingest month after month, the more likely we will be to have to report additional death statistics to the drug companies. Do not think this could not happen to you.

Now before you panic, let me assure you that the news isn't all bad. There is a way to lower the risks of these events we've talked about happening to you or your family. It begins with educating yourself about the dangers lurking in those little white bags and, even more important, learning how to structure your life so that you'll need to take fewer—if any—dangerous drugs in the future. That's the purpose of this book: to arm you with the information you need to keep your medicine cabinet from turning into a chamber of horrors.

## Are You in Jeopardy?

If you stopped reading this book right now, you would be in jeopardy of doing something that could be equally as dangerous as not acknowledging this serious issue—that is, shunning medications altogether. That would be a mistake. Let me emphasize this: *There is a place for modern medicine. There is a place for those little white bags. There is a place for doctors and scientists and people who work for drug companies—most of whom are more altruistic than we might think.* I prescribe drugs—powerful and potentially dangerous drugs—on a daily basis. But it behooves me and my patients *and you* to understand the risks and learn what is acceptable and what is not. In today's world this is quite a challenge. There does not seem to be a reliable, unbiased source of complete information to help you lower the risk of these tragedies happening to you.

Having blind faith in pharmaceuticals is more than just dangerous—it's naive. Why would we ever think that medications can cure illnesses that develop as the result of a lifetime of bad habits? Why would we look to a pill or a potion to dig us out of the physical or mental hole we've been digging, sometimes for decades? Although this may come as a shock to some people, we don't have high cholesterol because our bodies are low on statins. Our blood doesn't have the consistency of salad dressing because we haven't been taking expensive blood thinners. We're not overweight for lack of diet pills. I have never seen someone with type 2 diabetes cured by a medication. The fact is, if we don't have a healthy immune system, an antibiotic will not cure a bacterial infection. Sometimes we're sick because for many years we've lived unhealthy lifestyles and thought we could get away with it. Sometimes we are sick because our broken society all too often places profits over propriety. Sometimes we're sick because we have an unwavering belief that modern medicine can cure anything.

The truth is, modern medicine cannot even cure the common cold. At best, modern medicine can help keep us alive long enough for the results of some other bad habit to finish us off. We as a society are out of control when it comes to the appropriate use of medication. We must do something about the deaths. I do not want to read about one more Michael Jackson, Heath Ledger, or Whitney Houston. Equally important, I do not want to read about you or your family. People don't think these things we've talked about could happen to them, but let me tell you from firsthand experience, they are happening at staggering rates.

There is a way to live a longer, healthier, and more fulfilling life without opening yourself up unnecessarily to the inherent dangers of medications. That is why I'm writing this book. I want to provide a warning and then offer a viable, time-tested solution. Politicians talk about gun control, terrorist attacks, and traffic fatalities. That is all well and good. But it is time for everyone, including policy makers, to start talking about how medications are perhaps killing more people than guns, terrorists, and accidents. As you read on, the limited available statistics coupled with logic and personal experience will convince you. It is my hope and goal that this book will awaken the world and be a call to action. What I say in this book will not win me any popularity contests, but the information in it can change your life forever. I do not want a medication mishap for you.

# 3

# MEDICAL MISTAKES

*It is easy to get a thousand prescriptions but hard to get one remedy.*
—CHINESE PROVERB

Mrs. Young is a hardworking, eighty-year-young woman. She reminds me of my grandmother, energetic and feisty. In fact, she still works at a bakery in the town where I practice. Some time ago, she felt poorly early in the day but still managed to go to work, where the aroma of fresh bread and the sound of churning mixing bowls were ever present. Her doctor had given her a medication to help her blood pressure, and it had been doing the job for years. Mrs. Young had been told that the medication would help to make her heart stronger, so when she felt fatigued that morning, she reasoned that it must be her heart that was making her tired and that if her medication was supposed to make it stronger, she should take another pill. She would surely feel less tired if her heart were beating stronger. But Mrs. Young did not realize that the medication, known as a beta-blocker, worked by slowing down her heart rate.

After an hour or so at work, she felt even more tired. Reasoning that two pills would accomplish twice as much as one would, she took two more pills. A little while later she nearly passed out, and helpful coworkers rushed her to the emergency room. There the heart monitor indicated that her pulse rate was in the low thirties. Normally her heart rate ran in the fifties. The medication had slowed her heart rate. Medication was given to reverse the effects of the beta-blocker overdose, and Mrs. Young's heart rate began to speed up. The real cause of her extreme fatigue turned out to be dehydration.

Mrs. Young was fortunate. If she had not been at work, the outcome might have been much different. How many other people make similar mistakes with less-fortunate outcomes?

Could something like this happen to you? Lately, I have seen more and more of this happening. People are human. People misunderstand. People make mistakes. And as aging occurs, people make mistakes more frequently. This type of medical mistake can end in death. Medicines can kill in a variety of ways, including adverse reactions, misuse, and deadly interactions with other medications. However, medical mistakes are all too common and frequently are not reported or even realized, especially in the elderly, when it's easy to assume that death resulted from natural causes. Mrs. Young made an honest mistake. It is sad to say, but as our population ages—and this includes you and me—there will inevitably be more and more symptoms. Parts wear out. With more and more symptoms will come more and more prescriptions for medicines. The mistakes as well as deaths from mistakes will increase exponentially. These mistakes are made at various levels. Let me explain.

Mistakes can be made in the production and packaging of a medication. Mistakes can be made by the pharmacies that dispense the billions of pills yearly. Doctors, nurses, and caregivers can make mistakes. And so can patients. Just ask Mrs. Young. She admits she made a mistake. She lived and learned. Others are not as fortunate.

A landmark article titled "Death by Medicine," published in 2003, when fewer prescriptions were being written, gives us a glimpse into the serious problem of medical mistakes. Remember, most mistakes are never recognized or reported. The Institute of Medicine in 2000 estimated a very low number—98,000 deaths a year—from medical errors of all sorts.[1] In 1997, Dr. Lucien Leape estimated the medical- and drug-error rate at three million, with an annual fatality rate of 420,000.[2] Granted, this also includes medical errors, but can you imagine the magnitude of the problem as more and more prescriptions are written for a myriad of symptoms? These figures represent documented deaths from mistakes. In this same article, researchers Lazarou and Suh estimate 106,000 deaths annually from adverse drug reactions in the hospital.[3] Still others estimate 199,000 deaths from outpatient drug reactions a year. If you add up the deaths from adverse drug reactions in hospitals and outpatient deaths from adverse drug reactions alone, this comes to approximately 300,000 deaths a year. If we add Leape's medical-error data from 1997 (420,000) to the adverse-drug-reaction data, we have 720,000 deaths a year. If we factor in the many more prescriptions written now along with the aging population and overworked health care teams, the numbers are staggering. Sad to say, but I believe this represents just a fraction of the actual deaths that are occurring from medications. As you will see, besides the adverse reactions and mistakes for which we have a plausible number from years ago, many of the other ways medications are killing are just not recorded. The number of 720,000 deaths a year is significant, much higher than those from cardiovascular disease, statistically the number one cause of death.

It is not popular in the medical profession to talk about mistakes, so I give Dr. Leape a great deal of credit. In an article in the *Journal of the American Medical Association*, he opened the discussion of medical error.[4] It is now time to continue this discussion as well as to suggest solutions.

In Dr. Leape's article, he admitted that the literature on medication error leading to death is sparse. I believe that is an understatement. As you read on, you will understand why.

## A Death Is a Death

If a car bomb goes off in Afghanistan, we know about it the same day it happens. If a student spills her lunch on the president of the United States, the world knows in minutes. Television, radio, Facebook, and Twitter make the dissemination of news easy (and often annoying). Information regarding medication error, however, is vastly underreported. And yet the truth is, a death is a death.

Doctors continue to say they need more studies before they can support changing the culture of medicine. But there just are not enough studies or public reporting of medical mistakes, nor will there be. If the media had to give proportionate coverage to every death, regardless of the cause, we would begin to see the magnitude of the problem. Of course, that is not the case. But I hope that by the time you finish reading this book, you will realize that this problem, which is underappreciated, underreported, and misunderstood, belongs to everyone. We can be individually responsible.

## Mistakes Made in Production

My eyes were stinging from suppressed tears as I heard the story of a young woman who had died of cardiac arrest. She was taking a medication for atrial fibrillation, an abnormal heart rhythm where the top chambers beat faster than the lower chambers. The medication was supposed to suppress the rhythm. She had been on this medication for years without any problem whatsoever. Then, suddenly, her heart just stopped.

A week after her death, a notice was sent by the manufacturers, notifying patients on this medication that there had been an error, and they might have received a much higher dose of the medication than had been prescribed. The pills contained double the amount of medication written on the package. Can you imagine how the woman's family felt? Was it possible that their loved one received a wrong dose and this contributed to her cardiac arrest? Mistakes are made at many different levels. And, yes, they occur during production.

Just a few years ago there were reports of a contaminated blood thinner, heparin, which authorities believed originated in China. This contaminated medicine killed several people and caused serious problems in others. Something went awry in the production process. When I write a prescription, I now know that about 40 percent of pharmaceuticals are manufactured outside the United States. In addition, nearly 80 percent of the active ingredients used to make all our many medications come mainly from China and India. The Food and Drug Administration (FDA) has enough problems regulating medications made in the States. Who is making sure that the active ingredients are correct and are actually being placed in the medications I prescribe? Can you begin to imagine the problems we do not even know about? It makes me cringe.

Then there are counterfeit medications. Not long ago the *New York Times* reported,

Chinese government authorities have detained nearly 2,000 people as part of a nationwide crackdown on the sale of fake or counterfeit drugs and health care

products, according to a report on Sunday from
Xinhua, the official news agency. The government
said that . . . officials had seized about $183 million
in fake medicine, including fraudulent drugs for the
treatment of cancer, hypertension, and diabetes. . . .
The recent crackdown comes because of concern
that some of the fake medications are leading to liver
damage and even cardiac arrest.[5]

If two thousand were detained, how many more worldwide
are involved in this type of activity that leads to deaths from
the fake medications? This number must be added to the
total of medications that kill.

I support a global market, but the global market must be
inspected and regulated for quality. How can we know our
trust is not being broken by a supplier in China, a counter-
feiter in India, or an importer from somewhere else, not to
mention the fifteen-year-old on the assembly line in China
who simply makes a mistake? Many people believe the FDA
has the authority to monitor our imported drug supply; this
is not the case. Inspections in the US average every other year
for domestic pharmaceutical facilities. The FDA developed a
list of foreign facilities to aid in prioritizing inspections, but
it has been estimated it would take approximately nine years
to inspect the more than 3,500 facilities on this list just once.
And according to the same report, 64 percent of these may
never have been inspected.[6]

As I see funds for health care running low and the number

of prescriptions rising every year, the problem of contaminated, counterfeit, corrupted, and possibly mislabeled medicines is a real issue. I am concerned that the number of deaths from this type of production mistake will continue to rise and be unreported.

How do you know the medication you order on the Internet is not counterfeit? I want you to realize that mistakes are made in the production process. This includes labeling and packaging mistakes. As funding for monitoring production becomes sparse and as more and more prescriptions are written, it only is reasonable to assume that more and more fatal mistakes will be made. It takes funding to have early warning systems, educational programs, organizational system changes, and standards at every level in the production and distribution process. In a debt crisis do you actually believe this can happen? Unfortunately, production mistakes are not the only kind.

## Mistakes Made by Providers

The transition had been difficult from living independently to being watched and cared for by people Mrs. Davis didn't know. But now she was settling in to the nursing-home routine, and the sights and sounds swirling about her had taken on an almost soothing tone.

She was making new friends and getting to know the people behind the smiles as skilled men and women went about the task of caring for those who needed attention.

One night, Mrs. Davis began to feel "under the weather," as she told the staff. A virus that was passing through the facility had taken up residence in her body and was causing a growing degree of distress. Before long, she couldn't hold anything down and was suffering from debilitating diarrhea. For years Mrs. Davis had been on a diuretic to remove fluid from her body.

Because of her weakened condition, she couldn't eat or drink, but the staff was faithful in seeing that she received the prescribed medications day after day—including the diuretic, which was removing fluid from her body.

The combination of the body's natural response to most viral attacks—diarrhea and vomiting (the body's attempt to quickly flush out the attacker)—coupled with the constant administration of pills that further reduced the fluids in her system sent the suffering woman into acute dehydration. Before long, her kidneys failed, and Mrs. Davis died.

No one had intended to hurt her. No one had decided that she had lived long enough and it was her time to go. The simple, heartbreaking fact was that her worn and fragile body couldn't take the loss of fluids triggered by the infection and compounded by the endless stream of pills. She didn't die of the virus.

Bill went into a diabetic coma one night. Even though he was unaware of his surroundings, he kept receiving his diabetes medicine as his food and water intake plunged. When he became dehydrated, his kidneys and liver failed to break down his medications as efficiently as usual, and a 10-mg dose became the equivalent of a 50-mg dose. His blood sugar plummeted, and he became comatose from the low blood sugar, or hypoglycemia. Before long, he breathed his last, slipping away with his body undermined by the very medications that were supposed to have kept him alive.

Frances was on a blood thinner called Coumadin. She was frail, unsteady on her feet, and barely able to function. She also found it hard to sleep, so one night she was given a new sleeping pill. Shortly after, the woman went wild, stumbling down the hallway and slamming into people and potted plants. She fell and hit her head, causing internal bleeding, which sent her blood pressure plunging. Frances died.

Mistakes are made by medical personnel. Mistakes are made in pharmacies. Mistakes are made when someone misreads doctors' illegible handwriting. Mistakes are made by nurses. These mistakes can run the gamut from giving the wrong medication to a patient to giving the wrong dosage of the correct medication to failing to recognize when a medicine could do great harm because of a patient's dangerous condition.

Patients with kidney conditions or liver problems are at a greater risk than others. Providers can fail to alter a dosage to compensate for a patient's reduced kidney or liver function. Remember, these organs are responsible for breaking down medications.

Providers have reported fatal overdoses of the chemotherapy drug cisplatinum due to labeling similarities with carboplatin. Methotrexate, a medication used for arthritis and psoriasis, and also a form of chemotherapy, has been overdosed by inadvertent daily administration instead of weekly use. Fatal events from overdoses of magnesium sulfate, sometimes used to treat preterm labor, have been reported. Recently in a letter to health care professionals, the manufacturers of morphine sulfate, a commonly prescribed pain medication, have reported fatal overdoses when oral solutions were ordered in milligrams (mg) and then inadvertently misread and given as milliliters (ml). These are just a few of the many reported mistakes. Most mistakes go unreported or undetected.

---

### COMMON MEDICAL ERRORS

- Dispensing an incorrect or inappropriate dose
- Prescribing medications inappropriate for the medical condition
- Failure to monitor side effects
- Failure to communicate clearly with patients

---

Dr. David Phillips, in the journal *Pharmacotherapy*, has noted a spike in fatal medication errors at the beginning of each month. Because government checks are released at the beginning of the month, patients can afford to get their prescriptions filled. The increased pharmacy workload from this monthly surge in the sheer number of prescriptions increases pharmacy error rates, resulting in more fatalities.[7] Yes, pharmacists make mistakes.

Phillips also reported in the *Journal of General Internal Medicine* that a significant spike in fatal medication errors occurs inside teaching medical institutions during the month of July, when thousands of new medical residents start on-the-job training. He concludes that the July increase in mortality seen in his study results at least partly from changes associated with the arrival of new medical residents.[8] Yes, doctors make mistakes.

If you were able to add up accurately the mistakes made in production and the mistakes made by providers at every level, there would be some surprises. These are not purposeful mistakes. These are mistakes that human beings can make when their workload gets beyond a certain level.

## Mistakes Made by Patients

This brings us to the subject of patients' mistakes. In a study published in the *Archives of Internal Medicine* in 2000, 76 percent of the patients studied took their medications incorrectly.[9]

When placed in circumstances where a thorough reading of prescription information is expected, patients who have difficulty reading or cannot read at all might offer excuses such as "I don't have my glasses with me" or "I'll take it home and read it later." When filling out a form at the doctor's office, they might check every box on the patient history form in order to avoid detection and embarrassment. This places the provider in a position to make erroneous choices.

Some patients are so skilled at hiding illiteracy that their providers either assume that the patients are not taking their medicine as prescribed or conclude that the medication is not working. So they prescribe a higher dose.

Researchers from Vanderbilt University found that one-half of all heart patients made at least one mistake related to medicines after leaving the hospital. These patients knew about their conditions, had an attentive medical team, and had all their questions answered before being discharged. The study showed that 2 percent of the mistakes patients made were life threatening. This gives a glimpse into the magnitude of the problem. I suspect that in most medical situations, even more mistakes are being made.[10]

The stress of getting a new diagnosis also impairs patients' ability to follow through when medicines are prescribed. Patients will rarely admit that they don't understand something. They'll nod their heads as if what the doctor is saying is clear to them and they understand what the doctor means. In some cases, I presume, they simply don't want to know the truth and figure that not knowing what they need to know will keep whatever they fear from happening. They'll nod in agreement when told to take a certain pill three times a day, even though they may not fully understand the instructions and why it's important that they comply. They might not know the difference between a teaspoon and a tablespoon, figuring a spoon is a spoon. They might not realize that a tablet and a pill are the same thing.

Certain communication issues might exist even in

patients who do fully understand. For example, the doctor might say, "If you take this medication with your medicine for impotence, there could be problems." The patient hates being impotent, so knowingly goes against medical advice and bypasses the new prescription altogether. I've seen it happen far too many times.

Sometimes, it's what the *doctor* doesn't know that creates a problem with a medication. I heard one story about a physician who told his patient to take a pill—one designed to slow his heart rate—with each meal, assuming that his patient ate three meals a day. But this patient ate six meals a day, sometimes more, and was getting double or more the prescribed amount of medicine.

One gentleman thought the word *hypertension* meant he was "too tense." So he added an ample dose of over-the-counter tranquilizers and a soothing measure of alcohol to his prescribed blood pressure medications.

As you can see, patient mistakes are not necessarily related to recreational users looking for a chemical high and abusing prescription medicines to obtain it.

Health care professionals need to develop strategies to recognize this problem and ask patients to explain, in their own words, what was just said. But here again is a problem. As doctors' offices get busier and busier and as the population ages, we will see more and more people dying from medication mistakes simply because they didn't understand what they were supposed to do. And these mistakes don't take into account all those over-the-counter medications some

+

**FIVE QUESTIONS THAT WILL IMPROVE PATIENT LITERACY**

- Why am I taking this medication?
- How and when do I take this medication?
- What are the side effects, especially the dangerous ones?
- When should I not take this medication?
- What should I do if I forget to take this medication?

For more on health literacy go to www.health.gov/communication.

+

people mindlessly dump down their throats each day. People assume that since these medications are sold without a prescription, they are safe and carry little risk. This is just not true. I have seen cold medications and energy drinks cause fatal arrhythmias.

These types of situations and their resulting complications and deaths rarely show up in statistics. Patients' lack of understanding is just another way medications can kill. Let's take a closer look at the danger of not understanding medication instructions.

## Comprehending Instructions

I heard a story of a twenty-six-year-old woman who was crying outside her obstetrician's office.

"What's the matter?" another patient asked.

"I'm pregnant with my fourth child," the weeping woman shared between sobs. "I insert the birth control pills every day, and they just don't seem to be working."

Literacy in health care is more than just being able to read. It includes the ability to comprehend instructions well enough to act on them correctly. The 2002 report on the results of the National Adult Literacy Survey estimated that between 40 and 44 million Americans could not read at all or read at only a very basic level. An additional 50 million were found to be marginally literate. This adds up to 90 million people.[11] Some of these people are taking medicines that can kill if not taken correctly.

I, like most cardiologists, frequently prescribe the blood thinner Coumadin. This medicine helps treat and prevent blood clots. It also literally scares me every time I write a prescription for it. If patients do not take this medication correctly, their blood could quickly become too thin or too thick. If the blood is too thin and patients were to bump their heads, the fragile arteries could start to bleed, and clotting would not occur. The bleeding wouldn't stop.

If the blood is too thick, an oversized clot could form and block the flow of blood, causing major problems. This clot could break free and travel to other parts of the body, causing blockages in the brain, the lungs, the heart, or other vessels—all of which can be fatal.

Among minorities, it's estimated that two out of five adults read below the fifth-grade level.[12] The elderly are at even greater risk. They scored, on average, an entire reading level lower than young or middle-aged adults who could read. The problem is made worse by age-related challenges in hearing, memory, attention span, energy level, and communication skills. Our population is aging, and these aging individuals are the ones who are taking the most medications.

Many functionally literate patients (those who read at or below the fifth-grade level) have problems, too, because most health care material is written on a tenth-grade level or higher. A significant number of patients can't decipher the instructions on the label. Also, most doctors talk to the patients on a much higher plane than they can understand. One study of Medicare patients with chronic diseases found that 24 percent had inadequate health literacy about their diseases and 12 percent had only marginal functional literacy.[13] That makes up 36 percent of Medicare patients—over one-third! These patients never show up in the statistics.

But before we lay the blame on the sagging shoulders of the sick, let me assure you that the medical profession shares much of that particular load.

One of my partners told me of a patient who had Coumadin toxicity. As I mentioned before, Coumadin is probably the most dangerous medication I prescribe. It's used to lower the risk of blood clots by thinning the blood and allowing it to pass through restricted areas of damaged arteries. The use of this medication must be monitored closely. A fall, a wound, or a ruptured blood vessel can very quickly turn into a catastrophe. A bleeding stomach ulcer can't be stopped. A broken hip, a nosebleed, or "leaking" lungs can become lethal if the blood will not clot because of the Coumadin effect.

This patient had been told to take 3 mg of Coumadin once a day. For whatever reason, this patient was taking 3 mg of Coumadin *three times a day*. Blood tests showed, not surprisingly, that her blood was dangerously thin. The simplest injury could have proven deadly. I'm thankful to be able to say that this lady survived. Others aren't as fortunate.

This is not an isolated problem. With doctors having less and less time to spend with patients, and patients not being diligent (or having help) to protect themselves from mistakes, such situations are becoming more and more frequent. Add patients' mistakes to the list of ways in which medications can kill.

---

+

---

### TOP FOUR CONCERNS OF PATIENTS TAKING PRESCRIPTION MEDICATIONS

- Desired more detailed information about the benefits of the medication
- Wanted more specific information on adverse reactions
- Needed specifics on dosing and timing of dosing
- Concerned about getting prescriptions from multiple specialists with limited access to the prescribing physicians as well as limited access of the specialists to one another.

---

+

---

## Real Solutions

What I'm trying to say here is that we have a very real problem. Until the educational system of this country starts producing students who can actually read well, until pharmaceutical companies ramp up their quality control, until providers—including doctors—learn how to talk to their patients as opposed to over their heads, and until patients refuse to leave the physician's office until they fully understand what they're supposed to do, the problem will only get worse.

The truth is, you are part of the solution. After all, it's *your* body into which you may be about to pour a potentially dangerous chemical. It's *your* mind that can become clouded as a result of taking a particular medication. While under the influence of certain drugs, you may not be able to drive or think "right," and yet you may find yourself in situations where mental acuity is needed for survival. As you listen to your doctor, embrace the truth about your condition, and accept his or her suggested treatments with firm determination instead of fear. Write things down in your own language, and have your doctor check your facts.

Perhaps better yet, you can lower the risks of exposure to these mistakes we discussed by changing your lifestyle. This might alter your body's chemistry to the point where a prescription is unnecessary and the inherent risk of mistakes somewhere in the process is lower. Learn to take charge of your own health. Begin working to undo what you've been doing over the years, and begin striving to heal from the inside out, not the outside in. We'll talk more about this in later chapters.

# 4

# ADVERSE REACTIONS AND INSUFFICIENT RESEARCH

*He's the best physician that knows the worthlessness*
*of the most medicines.*
—BEN FRANKLIN

IF YOU WANT to scare yourself into a cardiac event, read the side-effects section that came with your latest prescription drug. Or, better yet, visit the over-the-counter section at your local drugstore or grocery store and browse through the "warnings" issued with such popular medications as aspirin or those "proven effective" sleeping pills. Several of these "safe" medicines list sudden death as a possible adverse reaction to their use. *Sudden death?*

When I was a third-year medical student, I was definitely at the bottom of the totem pole. It was my job to tag along behind the attending physician, the fellows, the residents, the interns, and the fourth-year medical students. If you watch medical dramas, you've probably seen images of this lab coat–clad entourage wandering across your television screen from time to time. All of us bottom-feeders were hoping to learn something from anyone who was willing to give us the time of day.

One fall afternoon, our attending physician stopped to console a family in the emergency room. I later found out that this young couple had a six-year-old son who had been suffering with asthma. The child had contracted a strep throat infection and had received penicillin—a common and well-tested antibiotic—for the infection.

Within minutes, the boy's body revolted. They rushed their son to the emergency room, but despite all that modern medicine had to offer, the professionals could not save their young patient from the immediate effects of the antibiotic. The boy died.

I was terribly shaken. As I watched the attending doctor console the family, I looked down the long, uncertain path of my own future career. Would I have to worry the rest of my life that each time I wrote a prescription, this could be the outcome? Would I have to worry about circumstances over which I had no control? Would part of my job description include the constant checking of the organs that broke down the medications I prescribed so those drugs didn't stay too long in the body and become more toxic than helpful? Would I have to constantly be reading and learning about new medications? Would I have to spend sleepless nights wondering whether I had killed or was killing patients who had trusted me with their lives? Was I getting information about medicines from agencies with questionable priorities?

And finally would I, *could* I, be the one who said, "I think this is too risky," when my patients were bombarded by the media, their friends, other doctors, and passionate relatives, urging them to take the latest and greatest medication?

The answers to those questions began to formulate in my mind that autumn day as I listened to the soft sobs of those grieving parents. Yes, I *would* always be concerned. Yes, I *would* have to check and recheck my patients. Yes, I *would* come to realize that sometimes the battle to protect a life can be part of a very lonely war.

My profession is a two-edged sword. I'm trained to heal, yet the treatments I'm trained to use can inadvertently kill. That day I was introduced to one of the most dangerous drug-induced adverse reactions a person can experience: an anaphylactic reaction.

### Removal of Protection

The term *anaphylaxis*, coined by Paul Portier and Charles Richet in 1902, means "removal of protection." It's derived from the Greek words *ana* ("against"), and *phylaxis* ("protection"). This is not a medical textbook, so I won't go into the details of the physiology, but I do want you to know that triggering anaphylaxis is one of the ways medicines kill.

When foreign substances such as venom from a bee sting or snakebite, assorted poisons, or powerful drugs are introduced into the human body, a wide variety of substances from the immune system may become activated; sometimes right away, sometimes after a second exposure. Some of these substances can generate a host of deadly reactions, which may lead to cardio and respiratory collapse.

Other parts of the body, including the skin and gastrointestinal tract, can get involved as well. As the immune system attacks the foreign substance, biologic mediators including histamines, bradykinins, platelet-activating factors, leukotrienes, and many more are released. Let's make this simple. Think of all those substances with the long names as members of an army attacking an invader. Some act as foot soldiers, others as the artillery, some as intelligence officers, and some as messengers to recruit more soldiers to the fight. The ensuing battle can be described by the word *inflammation*. This leads to symptoms that may include simple itching; a rash; edema (swelling) involving the head and neck; dangerous spasms of the airway, making it difficult or impossible to breathe; debilitating cramps, in any muscle; and in some cases, complete cardiovascular collapse. Cardiovascular collapse refers to dropping blood pressure, out-of-sync heart rhythms, and even heart attack. Every organ system may be involved in this cascade of fatal reactions. Without sufficient blood pressure and oxygen in the cardiovascular system, the body perishes.

Can medications trigger this deadly reaction? The answer goes to the core of why drugs are dangerous. *All* medications have the potential to cause this reaction. Penicillin is the most common, but the list includes other antibiotics, aspirin, muscle relaxants, opioids, nonsteroidal anti-inflammatory drugs (NSAIDs), seizure medications, contrast agents ("dyes") used for diagnostic testing, and intravenous anesthetics, to name just a few.

## Limited Data

The obvious question is, How often does this type of reaction occur? The answer is hard to determine because other medical conditions such as sepsis (a toxic condition resulting from the spread of bacteria), heart attack, and respiratory failure can mimic an anaphylactic reaction. The data is limited, and reporting systems remain poor, although some countries—such as the United Kingdom, France, and Australia—do keep registries.

An article in the *Archives of Internal Medicine* reviewed the medical literature and came up with these conclusions: "The occurrence of anaphylaxis in the US is not as rare as generally believed."[1] It's estimated that one in 2,700 hospitalized patients suffers from an anaphylactic reaction. The risk of death is estimated to be about one percent, with as many as 500 to 1,000 deaths annually. Of the 1,500 reported deaths from anaphylaxis, 75 percent of fatal reactions in the United States were from penicillin.[2]

The authors concluded that the available estimates were greatly underreporting the problem. I agree. Not all emergency departments, hospitals, or doctors report anaphylaxis. And what about those people who self-medicate or take over-the-counter medications and suffer the reaction?

There is not a system in place to properly obtain the real data regarding deaths from anaphylaxis. There is also a myriad of reasons not to report the problem. Fear of the legal system, lack of profits, and determining who is going to pay for what drive the silence. The bottom line is, we have an underappreciated, underreported problem that kills. Allow me to construct a hypothetical scenario.

In October 2009, the *Journal of Clinical Allergy and Immunology* reported that in 1980 there were 21 anaphylactic reactions per 100,000 patients. In 1990 we can assume that number had increased to 50 in 100,000, essentially doubling in a ten-year span.

Now, what if we continued the trend and doubled that to 100 reactions in 100,000 patients in 2000? Then doubled it again ten years later in 2010? That would be 200 anaphylactic reactions in 100,000 patients. Now, observe the many new medications currently available and how we, as a drug-centered society, take more and more medications per person per year. The numbers, based on this assumption, would come out to 2,000 reactions per million and 600,000 anaphylactic reactions per 300 million. Assuming a one percent death rate from anaphylaxis as reported in the review article in the *Archives of Internal Medicine* cited earlier, that leaves us with 6,000 deaths a year from anaphylaxis.

If four airliners, each with one hundred passengers on board, went down each month, people would be talking. The Federal Aviation Administration (FAA) would be taking action. There would be legislation designed to end those tragedies. People would do a lot more driving or riding on buses and trains.

But here we are with anaphylaxis killing us in numbers far too large to ignore. And what are we doing about it? Very little. Why? Because those deaths are taking place within the "safe" boundaries of the medical profession.

Well, isn't it time for someone to say, "Enough is enough"? Isn't it time for patients to think twice about the possibility that their bodies may rebel against a medicine to the point of death? Isn't it time to start looking for a viable substitute for introducing an endless stream of drugs into our bodies?

You might think we'd know the answer to those questions. Think again.

## What Is an Adverse Reaction?

An anaphylactic reaction is an extreme adverse reaction. It is important to note once again that medications can help save lives as well as cause adverse reactions that can take lives. The World Health Organization (WHO) defines an adverse drug reaction as a "noxious, unintended, and undesirable effect that occurs as a result of doses normally used . . . for diagnosis, prophylaxis, and treatment of disease or modification of physiologic function."[3] According to T. R. Einarson in the *Annals of Pharmacotherapy*, an average of 5 percent of reported hospitalizations were the result of adverse drug reactions.[4] Note the word *reported*. This study also was done in 1993 when the number of prescriptions written was much lower. The results of a Harvard study reported that 10 to 20 percent of hospitalized patients will have an adverse reaction.[5] These adverse reactions increase the risk of death nearly twofold—1.88 percent to be exact—according to an article in the *Journal of the American Medical Association* (JAMA).[6] It is well established that the more medications a patient is on, the greater the risk of an adverse reaction. A study published in the *Indian Journal of Pharmacology* demonstrated that this is a global problem, with .2 percent of total admissions ending in a death attributed to an adverse drug reaction.[7] Let's do the math. That equates to 2 deaths from adverse drug reactions in 1,000 hospital admissions, or 2,000 deaths in a million admissions. It is beyond the scope of this book to address the myriad of possible adverse reactions, but I do want you to be aware of the problem as I give examples of how adverse drug reactions are yet another way that medications can kill.

*Hormone Replacement Therapy*

For years, postmenopausal women have received hormone replacement therapy (HRT). The Women's Health Initiative Study, which evaluated the risks and benefits of hormone replacement therapy, was ended in 2002, when results of the study showed that women taking synthetic estrogen combined with synthetic progesterone had a higher incidence of ovarian cancer, breast cancer, stroke, and heart disease and little evidence of reduction in osteoporosis or the prevention of dementia.[8] In other words, the risks outweighed the intended benefits.

An article published in the British journal *Lancet* reported that the use of hormone replacement therapy in the United Kingdom over ten years in postmenopausal women resulted in an estimated additional twenty thousand breast cancers.[9] I have been unable to find American statistics for HRT in regard to an increase in breast cancer, stroke, uterine cancer, pulmonary embolisms, or heart attacks. The population in the States is roughly six times greater than that of Britain. There had to have been adverse reactions in the American group of people, leading to more deaths. Another example of an adverse reaction from a medication.

*Chemotherapy*

Chemotherapy is used in the treatment of cancer. Many providers feel that in cases of advanced cancer, chemotherapy may do more harm than good. It can trigger many adverse reactions, including killing the important bone-marrow cells, which make white blood cells that fight infection; red blood cells, which carry oxygen; and platelets, which help blood to clot. Chemotherapy can also damage other organs, including the heart, kidneys, and liver. Remember, an adverse reaction is an undesirable effect that occurs as a result of a normal dose. This can be thought of as a negative side effect when the reaction is small and not life threatening, but "negative side effect" is something of an understatement when the side effect or adverse reaction can take a life. Some time ago I had a patient whose heart muscle had been poisoned by chemotherapy. The

+

There are many stories about certain preexisting medical conditions altering the way a medication works in the body. If these conditions are not accounted for during the prescribing process, the outcome could be bad.

## CONDITIONS PREDISPOSING PATIENTS TO ADVERSE REACTIONS

- Dehydration
- Bleeding
- Alcohol use
- Sleep apnea
- Visual problems
- Obesity
- Addictions
- Kidney and liver disease
- Infections
- Advanced age

Why are older individuals more likely to have an adverse drug reaction? As people age, they generally have less water per pound of weight. Since doses are calculated on the basis of weight, once the amount of water in the body decreases, the concentration of the drug per pound of body weight will generally be higher in an older adult. Here are some other reasons:

- The liver is not as efficient in ridding the body of medications.
- The kidneys have decreased ability to clear drugs from the body. By age sixty-five, the filtering ability of the kidneys has already decreased by 30 percent. Other aspects of kidney function may also decline.
- Older individuals have a decreased ability to maintain blood pressure, and yet blood pressure medications are more risky to use as the body ages. Postural hypotension is a sudden fall in blood pressure when standing. If the body cannot compensate quickly when this happens, a fall could occur and a dangerous fracture could result. This is seen frequently in life-threatening hip fractures.

- Older individuals have less ability to adjust to very high and very low temperatures. Some medications can interfere with temperature regulation. The deaths of the elderly during heat waves or prolonged cold could be attributed to medications that interfere with a body's ability to control its temperature.
- Older individuals have more diseases. An older person may have a bad heart, kidney, or liver, thus increasing the chance of an adverse event.
- In the elderly the testing of drugs is often inadequate. In fact, most drugs are not tested in the elderly.
- The elderly are usually taking more medications, again increasing the risk of an adverse event.

---

+

---

chemotherapy had to be stopped. The heart did not recover from the toxic exposure to the chemotherapy.

In 2003, one study found that high-dose chemotherapy with stem-cell transplantation showed no significant benefit when compared with monthly conventional chemotherapy, and yet this type of treatment is used when conventional therapy has not worked.[10] The point is that chemotherapy might be worth the risk, but this class of medications is toxic and has severe adverse effects. Again, the concept of risk management must be evaluated for each individual. Is the risk worth the benefits? The adverse reactions associated with chemotherapy are significant.

### Psoriasis

Psoriasis is a chronic skin condition that leaves raised patches of scaly or inflamed skin. No one is sure what causes this condition. And although some think the body attacks itself, it is not a deadly condition. Efalizumab, a medicine that suppresses the immune system, was once used to treat psoriasis.

Unfortunately, this raised the risk of progressive multifocal leukoencephalopathy (PML). To state it simply, this is a disease caused by a common virus that is latent, or inactive, until the body's immune system is suppressed. Then the virus, now unopposed, inflames the white matter of the brain, destroying parts of the brain and causing a host of problems, including weakness, paralysis, blindness, and eventually death. Psoriasis is a non-life-threatening condition. But the medication once prescribed to treat it caused a life-threatening condition.

### Other Medications

Anticholinergics are medications that block a chemical called acetylcholine. They can be found in medicines used to treat depression, incontinence, and glaucoma. There can be many adverse reactions, including dementia.

An article in the *Journal of Psychiatry* reported on six patients who developed "intense, violent suicidal preoccupation after 2–7 weeks of fluoxetine treatment."[11] Certainly suicide would count as an adverse reaction.

In 1846, William Morton, a Boston dentist, changed the landscape of medicine with perhaps the most important innovation ever, anesthesia. This innovation ushered in the era of modern surgery. As I mentioned earlier, I grew up with a father who used these potentially toxic agents on a daily basis. The exact mechanism of many anesthetic agents is not well known. There are possible adverse reactions that could be fatal. These might include an oxygen deficiency if a patient does not breathe well as a result of the anesthetic medication, inhalation of stomach contents into the lungs in the event the patient vomits while unconscious, or a critically high fever caused by the medication, which can be life threatening. Anesthesia helps to save lives, but its use may also trigger adverse, sometimes fatal, reactions.

Remember, adverse reactions are possible with any medication. Most are not fatal, but any medication, whether an antibiotic, a chemotherapy drug, a blood thinner, a medicine to treat abnormal heart rhythms, a seizure medication, or a medicine used to treat the mind, can have fatal adverse reactions. The ultimate goal for each one of us is to minimize exposure to risk from medications and to recognize adverse effects early. I will explain how we can accomplish this a bit further down the road.

## Breakdown

A medication once sold under the name Baycol was designed specifically to help lower cholesterol. Anyone suffering from heart disease is concerned about cholesterol levels, so when this new "super" statin was released in 1997, I began prescribing it, hoping it would help my patients lower their risk of heart attack.

I checked liver functions routinely, as this medication was known to cause liver problems to develop. I also watched for a side effect called myositis. This is a muscle breakdown and can occur in one in one thousand statin users.

The drug worked as promised. Cholesterol levels dropped, and I assumed the risk-to-benefit ratio was similar to other statins. I was wrong.

Soon, the FDA issued a statement that the drug had been linked to thirty-one known deaths due to a condition called rhabdomyolysis. This is a condition in which muscle is destroyed, and the waste material from that destruction ends up in the bloodstream. The kidneys, faced with the overwhelming amount of toxins now circulating in the blood, reach the end of their ability to clean the flow, and they tumble into failure.

By 2001, after more than fifty deaths worldwide and over a thousand reports of rhabdomyolysis, Baycol was removed from the market. I was fortunate. I didn't have to report any problems with Baycol.

However, the situation with this pharmaceutical highlighted a problem associated with all statin drugs. The millions of people taking these medications share a common risk: myositis and liver damage. The risk versus benefit must be carefully considered. The fact that some people take these drugs regularly and suffer no such side effects doesn't mean the drug is safe. It just means that those people are either very lucky or the time bomb hasn't gone off yet.

## Anti-Inflammatories

Do you remember the well-documented Vioxx tragedy? Many people worldwide suffer from joint pains and arthritis, so they reach for relief in the form of anti-inflammatory medications that may cause significant gastrointestinal side effects. Vioxx was marketed as an anti-inflammatory with fewer gastrointestinal side effects.

I still remember the many and growing reports of gastrointestinal bleeding and of heart attacks, some fatal, generated by the drug. By September 2004, Vioxx was yanked from the shelves of pharmacies around the world.

You'd think there would have been a collective sigh of relief from pain sufferers everywhere. Not in my office. I remember the uproar from patients who wanted to know if they really had to come off Vioxx.

A study published in 2005 stated that Vioxx may have caused as many as 140,000 cases of heart disease and as many as 56,000 deaths during the five years it was on the market.[12] The published study of 1.4 million patients showed that Vioxx, if given in low doses, increased the risk of heart disease by about 50 percent and, if given in high doses, increased the risk by 358 percent.[13] Not only Vioxx but the entire class of anti-inflammatory medications known as NSAIDs (nonsteroidal anti-inflammatory drugs) poses a risk of adverse reactions. These medications are frequently used to treat arthritis, the most common chronic degenerative disease that physicians encounter. I have never had a patient die from arthritis, but many have died from the complications of NSAIDs. The main adverse reactions are gastrointestinal bleeding and damage to the kidneys. Vioxx added heart disease to the list.

When I read this, I began to wonder if my main job as a cardiologist should be to keep people *off* medications unless they are at an acute stage in their illness and need it to extend life. Maybe, just maybe, they could learn to control their inflammation through dietary choices, moderate exercise, or the chemical-changing power of simply laughing more.

## Update on Vioxx

In 2011, the New York Times News Service reported the following:

> Merck has agreed to pay $950 million and has pleaded guilty to a criminal charge over the marketing and sales of the painkiller Vioxx, the company and the Justice Department said Tuesday.
>
> The negotiated settlement, which includes resolution of civil cases, was the latest of a series of fraud cases brought by federal and state prosecutors against major pharmaceutical companies.
>
> By the time Vioxx, which was approved by the Food and Drug Administration in 1999, was pulled off the market in 2004 because evidence showed that it posed a substantial heart risk, about 25 million Americans had taken the drug.

In a statement on Tuesday, Merck said that it had previously disclosed the seven-year investigation by the United States attorney in Massachusetts and had charged $950 million against its earnings in October 2010.

Merck agreed to pay a $321 million criminal fine and plead guilty to one misdemeanor count of illegally introducing a drug into interstate commerce, the Justice Department said in a news release. The charge arose from Merck's promotion of Vioxx to treat rheumatoid arthritis before the FDA approved it for that purpose in 2002. . . .

"When a pharmaceutical company ignores the F.D.A. rules aimed at keeping our medicines safe and effective, that company undermines the ability of health care providers to make the best medical decisions on behalf of their patients," Tony West, assistant attorney general of the Justice Department's civil division, said in a statement.[14]

As I read this article, several things jumped out at me. First, $950 million is a lot of money, which underlines the fact that money plays a role in this dilemma. If the makers of Vioxx did this—and got away with it for a time—how many other medications out there pose similar risks? What doctor has the time to go through the red tape and hassle of filing an adverse-drug report? Should doctors and their patients serve as guinea pigs when medicines are brought to market too quickly?

## Children at Risk

### *The Unborn*

Don't think for one minute that adverse reactions happen only in adult bodies. Some reading this book are blessed with children. But let's go back even further. Unfortunately, medications have killed and are killing the unborn as well.

Many adult medications can do great harm to those tiny forms of life hidden away inside their mothers' wombs. We call a medication that can do harm to the unborn a teratogen.

The first teratogen to which I was introduced in medical school was thalidomide. This medication, developed in Germany, was used to help battle the symptoms of morning sickness. But it soon became horribly obvious that this drug had affected the limbs and organs of more than eight thousand developing babies. We can be thankful that thalidomide never made it to the US market, although twenty thousand US patients did receive the drug as part of a clinical trial.[15] However, an awakening had occurred: developing babies in the womb can be just as vulnerable to medications as everyone else.

Follow me for a moment. Birth defects are the leading cause of infant mortality in the United States, accounting for 20 percent of deaths. Of all newborns, there is a 3- to 5-percent occurrence of birth defects. One thousand babies born means the potential for thirty to fifty birth defects.

It's estimated that 10 percent of all birth defects are related to exposure to a teratogenic agent, including medication.[16] Every time I see a woman of childbearing age as a patient, I have to look up the medications she is on.

In one study, 488,175 women ages 15–44 had 1,011,658 prescriptions filled. One out of six of these women received a drug that could cause birth defects![17] Medications can kill the unborn. These numbers need to be added to our running total.

This particular study also uncovered the fact that these women were no more likely to receive special counseling than those receiving far less risky medications. And these are the medications with adverse reactions we know about.

*Depression in Children*

Children are using prescription medications more and more. Years ago a child would rarely receive a medication. Today children are not only receiving antibiotics for infections at alarming rates, they are also receiving more and more medications for mental illnesses, including attention deficit disorder and depression.[18] Yes, depression. It is estimated that 4 percent of preschoolers suffer from depression. The diagnosis of depression in children has risen 23 percent.[19] With this rise in medication use, the adverse reaction rate will increase as well.

The standard antidepressant treatment is a class of

medications called selective serotonin reuptake inhibitors (SSRIs). There is considerable debate about whether this therapy is effective. But regardless of the mechanism, more and more children are receiving selective serotonin reuptake inhibitors. One of the possible adverse reactions to this class of medications is suicide. Are these children going to be on these medications for the rest of their lives?

## Emergency Call

Some time ago I received a call from an emergency room doctor. A patient who had undergone bypass surgery a year ago was back in the emergency room with pain along his incision line. He had been taking heavy narcotics since the surgery, trying to relieve his symptoms.

The physician knew him all too well, as he frequently came in needing intravenous medications for pain when his pills ran out. The ER doctor had chosen to prescribe an anti-inflammatory this time.

The patient's electrocardiogram, chest X-ray, and blood work were all normal. When his doctor administered medication to this fifty-nine-year-old, the patient experienced an anaphylactic reaction. His respiratory system collapsed, his blood pressure dropped, and in a very short period of time, he went from complaining of having pain along his incision to not being able to breathe.

The doctor responded with steroids, Benadryl, and epinephrine. Unfortunately, the epinephrine caused one of the man's coronary arteries to spasm and precipitated a heart attack. That's why the doctor called me.

This time, the story has a happy ending. The man survived. But his experience is reflective of a common and growing problem. Medicines kill even in tightly controlled environments, even with a doctor hovering over you, even with the full weight of modern medicine bearing down on the problem.

## OTCs

Don't point your finger just at prescription medications. Over-the-counter medications (OTCs) also can produce adverse events. Pharmaceutical giant Johnson & Johnson is reducing the maximum recommended daily dose of its pain reliever Extra Strength Tylenol to lower the risk of accidental overdosing. Acetaminophen? This little pill has been around for years! We can purchase it without a prescription. I can tell you one thing: livers—yes, livers—everywhere are safer because of that change.

The truth is, acetaminophen—not liver cancer, not hepatitis, not alcohol—is the top cause of acute liver failure.[20] It's found in many over-the-counter preparations. When most people pluck a cold medication from their local drugstore, they are not looking at the ingredients or even thinking about their livers. They are thinking about a stuffy nose or a headache or achy muscles. They just want relief. But too much acetaminophen can have adverse effects on the liver.

We also need to mention pseudoephedrine, the active ingredient in many cold medications. This is also the substance used to make methamphetamines. What? You mean I just took "speed" for my cold? Yes.

OTCs can have adverse reactions just as prescription medications can. Sometimes these adverse reactions can kill.

### Insufficient Research

Debbie came to the office with extreme shortness of breath and a fast heart rate. She could scarcely walk across the room without collapsing into a chair and gasping for breath. While some medical conditions can affect a person this way—especially someone well advanced in years—Debbie was only eighteen and was busy preparing for college.

A month earlier she'd been diagnosed with inflammation of the colon. Up to this point, she'd been the picture of health.

A new medication—a drug touted as a breakthrough in the treatment of her condition—had been prescribed, and Debbie had been taking it faithfully, confident that it would soon work its wonders and help her get on with her life.

As I listened to her history, I began putting two and two together. Her symptoms simply weren't the result of an inflamed colon. They had to be the result of her medication, a new drug about which I'd heard very little.

Later that day, I went to the patient information provided by the company that had created the drug and began to read, and everything began to fall into place. This new medication could cause *every* symptom Debbie had described. What alarmed me most was the fact that its makers had tested this medication on only a very small number of individuals before it had been brought to market.

Years ago many, many patients were part of testing before any new drug was released to the general public. These trials could last for years, and the drug's adverse reactions could be discovered and at least mitigated in some way. But, it seemed, times have changed. These days, so many medications aren't tested long enough to discover more than just a handful of their possible side effects.

It was Debbie's new medication that was wreaking havoc on her quality of life. I knew, beyond a doubt, that if she continued taking it, the reaction she was experiencing would soon become life threatening.

Speaking of life threatening, exactly when does a new medicine merit that label? Consider these facts based on a report of another new drug I recently researched: the study group consisted of almost sixteen hundred patients. Of these, one died in close temporal association with the drug. Does that mean if 16,000 patients took the medication, we'd be looking at 10 deaths? Carrying that forward just a little, if 160,000 people took the medication—a very low number in today's drug-saturated society—would 100 succumb? Would that be life threatening enough? If pharmaceutical history is any indication, the answer would be a polite but firm no.

My point is that no one really knows when enough is

enough, unless you happen to be a friend or relative of the person who gave his or her life in support of an industry that sometimes seems to care more about profits than about lives. How much are you willing to risk to find out whether the drug company got it right?

I know this sounds harsh. But having to lower a loved one's body into an early grave because a pharmaceutical company didn't do its homework and rushed a medicine to market is a harsh reality too.

## Dirty Little Secret

I am always extremely careful about prescribing a medication that has just been released to the public. There's a reason for this.

After the AIDS epidemic struck, with its devastating impact on the lives of thousands of people, it was determined that a medication was needed to fight the epidemic, and it was needed *now*. So a fast-track system to get medications approved was initiated. So many people were dying of AIDS that the old process of obtaining medication approval—working out the dangerous side effects, finding the right dosage levels, examining harmful multidrug interactions—was, in the minds of many, taking too long. Much of that testing traditionally took place far from our shores. It seems that those living in the United States were in the enviable position of benefiting from what a new drug did—for better or for worse—to those of other countries.

Before 1990, only 3 to 4 percent of medications were released first in the United States. After fast-tracking came into vogue, that percentage grew to what it is today: 66 percent of new drugs hit the American market right out of the starting gate.[21] That's right. We get to take that first ride down the track, holding on with all we've got, hoping against hope that what's under us will see us through. With all the money put into research and development, along with the incredibly high cost of marketing a new product, one can see why the owners of that product would want to get it into the bloodstreams of as many people as possible in as short a time as possible. In this environment, objectively evaluating the safety of a medication takes both time and resources. Also, to make matters worse, *USA Today* reported in September 25, 2000, that one-half of experts hired to evaluate drug safety by the government have conflicting interests. Who can afford that?

The fast track was implemented with the noblest of intent: get medications designed to save AIDS and cancer patients out the door ASAP. But it seems that suddenly our lives began to be threatened by everything from high blood pressure, an elevated cholesterol count, and even the stresses of everyday life. Suddenly, *everything* was out to do us in. Very quickly, we found ourselves falling victim to unproven products which, themselves, have become life threatening.

Today, post-marketing surveillance is the way medication safety is evaluated. I don't want my patients to be the ones exposed to this dirty little secret. I don't want those who come to me for healing to be strapped to a new medication like a medical crash-test dummy and sent down the highway of life to see if the claims of the drug industry will help them survive their first encounter with an immovable object. I'd much rather be prepared than surprised.

## Finding Hope

I recognize that even if we do everything perfectly, there will be problems with medications. That comes with the territory. However, it might be high time that we recognize there are better ways to change our bodies' chemistry. These methods need to be researched and marketed just as aggressively as the latest and greatest wonder drugs.

Instead of funding weight-loss pills, how about promoting weight-loss programs? Instead of sleeping pills, how about finding out why patients don't sleep well and getting at the cause rather than treating a symptom? Instead of medicating pain, let's find out what is causing the pain.

To turn this problem around, we individually—and collectively—need to recognize the problem, learn all we can, and discover ways to minimize medication's place in our lives. I don't think we can legislate this. And I don't think the system that currently exists can be easily reformed. No, this change must come one voice at a time. The real solution will reveal itself as we go back to the way we were originally designed and work to change our bodies' chemistry based on those parameters.

For now, when you're faced with a health issue—even one that is life threatening—don't place all your hopes on a wonder drug to see you through in the months and years to come. Instead, start searching for ways to heal the problem and find the reason why you are sick. Start developing a plan for healing that doesn't necessarily have to include those little pills and potions in those little white bags. Start looking for the ultimate healing that, in my experience, can be found in only one way of life. We'll talk more about this in later chapters.

# 5

# MISUSE OF MEDICATIONS

*Poisons and medicine are oftentimes the same substance
given with different intents.*

**—PETER LATHAM**

Matt was twenty-one and an up-and-coming college student. He'd just returned from a fraternity party where he'd been drinking alcohol and smoking marijuana, trying to soothe his nerves after a fight with his girlfriend.

Matt's parents were away for the weekend, and when he returned home, he wanted a medication to help him relax. He knew that his mother had some tranquilizers, so he went into his parents' bathroom and took, according to third-party reports, "several" of her pills.

Matt's body was found the next day. It was hypothesized

that the combination of alcohol and tranquilizers caused him to quit breathing.

This tragic yet all-too-familiar story illustrates a growing trend today: misuse of medications.

When physicians write drug orders, they take into account many variables, such as dosing based on patients' kidney function, detailed instructions on how to use the medication, and careful consideration of interactions with other drugs the patients may be taking. Prescriptions are given to specific people, with specific limitations, for specific ailments. Move outside those guidelines, and you open the door to disaster. Matt is proof of that.

## Pill Parties

Pill parties bring together young people who've collected drugs from various sources, including their own homes or local street corners. At these parties, copious amounts of alcohol are usually used to wash down the pills. What types of pills? Who knows? The young people haven't a clue. All the collected drugs are simply dumped into a hat, and the hat is passed around. The result of this form of "entertainment" is often a visit to a hospital emergency room or a trip to the local morgue.

## Self-Improvement

Sometimes drugs take the lives of people who are simply trying to better themselves.

Janet had gained a few extra pounds and knew her mother was taking a medication to stimulate her thyroid gland. Janet wanted to "speed up" her metabolism. She would sneak into her mother's cache of pills and take one or two when the bottle was mainly full so the pills wouldn't be missed.

One winter day, fighting a cold, Janet added a medication containing pseudoephedrine, thinking she'd kill two birds with one stone. The next thing she knew, her heart started beating out of control. When I saw her in the hospital and tried to treat the atrial fibrillation, I had a difficult time overcoming the medications in her body. It wasn't until days later that she told me what she'd been doing. I'm thankful that Janet had a complete recovery and learned a valuable lesson. But many people's stories don't turn out so well.

A pediatrician told me about a family who wanted to keep their baby quiet so they could get a good night's sleep. They gave the infant an adult dose of a sleeping pill. Sure enough, the baby didn't disturb them all night long. Unfortunately, the baby never woke up.

Jon was a college student getting ready to drive home for the holidays. It would be an all-night trip, and he was already tired from taking final exams. Friends suggested he take those pills advertised to keep people from dozing off. "They keep you awake and sharp," they encouraged. Perhaps the pills did, for a while. But sometime in the night, Jon lost his life in a car accident. The misuse of medications, both prescribed and over the counter, is another way in which medications are killing.

## Suicide

Mark was successful. He was editor of a local publication. He did volunteer work at his church. At forty-one years of age, he seemed to have a good life. Actually, he and his wife were having problems, but none of his friends knew he was "on the brink." He deliberately overdosed on medications and died. Should suicide be included in deaths from medications?

One article reported that in 2007, approximately 27,000 people died from unintentional overdoses.[1] This is the equivalent of losing a 150-passenger airplane every day for six months. If we add the intentional overdoses like Mark's to this number, we have another way in which medications are killing: misuse of medication.

## Dangerous Situations

Perhaps you've reasoned yourself into a dangerous situation. Perhaps you've gotten away with it . . . for now. And, yes, before I cast too many stones, even physicians are guilty of stretching that line between common sense and perceived need. I include these tragic instances in the hope that perhaps something will sound familiar to you.

A chronic narcotic-seeking patient waited until the end of the day to see a doctor. The physician, who'd been up the entire night and had already seen forty patients, was bone tired and just wanted to go home. Rather than evaluate the patient's pain, he simply wrote a prescription for narcotics and sent the visitor away, not realizing that he was the *fourth* doctor the patient had seen in five days. What happened after that is anyone's guess. The darkness of night often hides from view the results of many of the terrible mistakes we make during the day.

Sometimes people misuse medications to feel better. Sometimes they do so in a desperate attempt to escape from reality and cope with issues of guilt and shame over something in their lives.

## Is Misuse Poisoning?

A blog article written by Shari Roan of the *Los Angeles Times* caught my eye. In her December 20, 2011, column, Ms. Roan wrote,

> Ninety percent of poisoning deaths in the United States are caused by drugs, the federal government reported Tuesday. Drug poisoning deaths now outnumber traffic deaths as the leading cause of injury death in the country.
>
> The report, from the National Center for Health Statistics, points to misuse or abuse of prescription drugs as the driver of the upward trend in poisoning deaths. The number of deaths from opioid painkillers (such as morphine, hydrocodone and oxycodone) rose from 4,000 per year in 1999 to 14,800 in 2008.

Those deaths are more common among males, people ages 45 to 54, non-Hispanic whites, American Indians or Alaska Natives than among other groups, the report said. About three-quarters of the deaths were accidental, 13 percent were suicides and 9 percent were undetermined, it said.

Overall, there were 41,000 poisoning deaths in the U.S. in 2008, the latest year for which statistics are available.

Although a concerted public-health campaign has lowered the rate of traffic fatalities over the last three decades, a similar effort may be necessary to curb the trend of poisoning deaths, the authors of the report said.[2]

It would seem from the wording used in this report that *poisoning* is the correct word.

---------------------- **+** ----------------------

### A LITTLE CAN KILL A LITTLE ONE

According to the American Association of Poison Control Centers, in 2002 there were 2.4 million toxic ingestions. Many prescription and over-the-counter medications are included in this total. In many situations a single pill can have the potential to kill if taken by an infant. Sometimes a caregiver turns away for a few seconds. Sometimes toddlers go where they should not go. Visitors may drop pills on the floor. Someone may inadvertently leave a medicine bottle out where a child can reach it. Following are some medications that are dangerous to the young if ingested.

- **OXYCODONE AND HYDROCODONE.** Lortab, Percocet, and Vicodin are a few of the common names for these painkillers. These can suppress the respiratory system and cause an infant or a young child to quit breathing. One-half tablet of oxycodone can be lethal.
- **CALCIUM CHANNEL BLOCKERS.** There are many of these, including diltiazem, verapamil, amlodipine, and nifedipine, to name a few. These blood pressure and rhythm medications can drop the blood pressure and slow the heart as well as cause seizures.
- **ANTIDEPRESSANTS.** These drugs, including those sold under such names as Elavil, Zyban, and Wellbutrin, can cause seizures and unresponsiveness.
- **SALICYLATES.** These include aspirin and can cause nausea, vomiting, seizures, coma, and death. Oil of wintergreen, which smells so good, can attract an infant. One tablespoon of oil of wintergreen is the equivalent of eighty baby aspirins.
- **CAMPHOR.** Ingestion of camphor—the active ingredient of many medicines, including Vicks VapoRub and Ben-Gay, which is used to help sore muscles (and by some people to stop the itch of bug bites)—can cause the rapid development of seizures, delirium, and coma in infants.

The toll-free number for the Poison Control Center is 800-222-1222. Keep it near your phone, save it to your cell phone, and tape it to the door of your medicine cabinet.

+

## Great Pains

One of the largest misuses of drugs occurring now involves the taking of pain medications. I recently heard a story of a twenty-three-year-old battling an addiction to crack cocaine. His mother always feared he'd die in a drug deal gone awry. The sad truth is that her son did die after an overdose. But he didn't breathe his last in some dark alley with copious amounts of crack cocaine coursing through his veins. No, he died on his mother's couch, safely cloistered in her home, after he took medications prescribed for him by a local pain clinic and given to him at a nearby pharmacy. His mother said his death has been even more painful because it was medical professionals, not drug dealers, who doled out the narcotics and antidepressants that led to his overdose. When you're drugged up, thinking about what you are doing, not to mention taking a medication correctly, is next to impossible.

Reports released by the TennCare program in Tennessee, the state in which I practice, show a steady increase in narcotic use from 1.03 million claims in 2007, costing $33 million, to 1.28 million claims in 2011, which cost $48 million. It is hard for me to believe that people need all that pain medication—drugs that merely treat a symptom and not even a disease. And these are statistics from just one state in the Union. Imagine the numbers for the entire country! We have a misuse problem that is killing us from the inside out. As I think about the problem, I can picture all those currently behind the wheel of fast-moving cars, working in dangerous jobs with heavy equipment, or even writing prescriptions while impaired. Those thoughts make me doubly committed to never getting into that situation myself. *Somebody* out there needs to be clearheaded. According to the Centers for Disease Control, one in eight teens has misused prescription painkillers. I wish I could say these individuals all had good judgment and understood how to minimize their risks.[3]

## Mindless Dangers

I'm reminded of a story reported in the *National Post*. According to the report, a Canadian judge ruled that the extreme, mind-altering effects of Prozac, an antidepressant drug, played a major role in causing a fifteen-year-old boy to stab one of his best friends with a nine-inch kitchen knife.

Apparently the Winnipeg boy had a history of drug "experimentation" before the crime but never had acted so aggressively. It was only when he began taking doctor-prescribed Prozac that he dove off the deep end and became "irritable, restless, agitated, aggressive, and unclear in his thinking." The judge, blaming Prozac for the boy's actions, refused to try him as an adult and sentenced him to only ten months more than the two years he'd already served while awaiting trial.[4]

In 2001, a Wyoming jury ruled that the antidepressant drug sold under the name Paxil had caused a man to murder his wife, daughter, and granddaughter before killing himself. It is alleged that Eric Harris, one of the mass murderers in the infamous Columbine High School shooting, had also been taking an antidepressant drug at the time of the tragedy.

If certain antidepressants can trigger these types of actions in some users, what about other mind-altering medications that so many people ingest so freely? Could it be that we're setting ourselves up for tragedies of our own? A fearful thought!

## Aurora, Colorado

We seem to be hearing about similar tragedies more frequently than ever before. The recent tragedy in Aurora, Colorado, has stunned the nation. As I was writing this chapter, twelve people in a movie theater were killed at a late-night showing of a Batman movie, and more than fifty were injured. Why did an intelligent, educated young man unleash such carnage? We may never know for sure, but he was alleged to have been taking a prescription painkiller sold under the name Vicodin, although he did not suffer from chronic physical pain. Reportedly, he was experimenting with the mind-altering drug. I can tell you that if he was taking this medication, it played a role in the tragedy. Medications can change the chemistry of the entire body, including the area of the brain where reasoning occurs. Mix some mind-altering medications with susceptible genetics, add some brain changes from prolonged exposure to violence on the television or in theaters, not to mention hours on gaming systems where the entire goal is to kill, and you can see how the limbic system of the brain, which controls the stress chemistry, can overpower the prefrontal cortex, where reasoning takes place.

People can snap for many reasons. Misuse of medications such as painkillers is playing an important role and is altering the ability to reason and make good choices. In this way, medications are killing indirectly. As our society continues down this road, we can expect to see more and more people snap. With over 30 percent of those under age 20 taking at least one prescription drug in the last month, the problem will continue to grow.[5] Medications for attention deficit disorder, painkillers, medications for anxiety and depression, sleeping medications, appetite suppressants, and energy-boosting medications all change the brain's function. Our young people with developing minds were not designed for medications, watching hours of violence, and video simulators where killing becomes second nature. I can see how in this vulnerable scenario medications can contribute to a breaking point. There may not be hard data, but misuse of medications contributing to tragedies like the one in Aurora, Colorado, would have to be considered another way medicines are killing. Logic says this is plausible.

To our list of ways medications are killing, we must now add the deaths from medications altering the mind and triggering these types of tragic events. We also must not forget the traffic accidents and other fatal accidents stemming from altered minds and dysfunctional reasoning. The numbers are beginning to add up: we have previously given the numbers from medication errors in hospitals and outpatient settings. We have some numbers on anaphylaxis to add to the total. Add to these the deaths from mistakes in production and distribution; from patient mistakes; from mixing and matching drugs; from adverse reactions, whether liver failure caused by overuse of acetaminophen or fatal gastrointestinal bleeding from nonsteroidal anti-inflammatory medications; deaths from known effects of medications, such as fatal heart rhythms, even when medications are used correctly; and now deaths indirectly effected by altered brain chemistry. I believe that any logical thinker can conclude that, directly or indirectly, medications are the number one cause of death. What are we doing?

Officials are trying to address the escalating problem by passing bills that would require doctors and pharmacies to consult a controlled-substance database before writing a legal prescription or dispensing these medications. But who is going to pay for the database and the additional time needed to monitor and police the disbursements? The drug companies?

## Not Typical Abusers

The problem is that many of those taking pain medications for both physical and psychological pains are not typical abusers. These medications are not being dealt on the street. Users walk into pharmacies carrying legitimate prescriptions written by legitimate doctors and dispensed by legitimate pharmacists. To make the problem worse, the Internet is a well-entrenched source of these medications, with users often trading information on which doctors are an easy source or a good place to get "Roxys," the street name for Roxicodone, a fast-acting form of the painkiller oxycodone. What can be done when these "patients" are taking and distributing legal medications?

One patient I recently saw had injured his back in a car accident. He went to a pain clinic—a privately owned

+

## DO WE REALLY NEED THAT DAILY ASPIRIN?

On January 16, 2012, the *New York Times* News Service reported that nearly a third of middle-aged Americans regularly take a baby aspirin in the hope of preventing a heart attack or a stroke or of lowering their risk of cancer. The article quoted Dr. Alison Bailey, director of the Gill Heart Institute at the University of Kentucky, where I trained, as saying, "People don't even consider aspirin a medicine, or consider that you can have side effects from it. That's the most challenging part of aspirin therapy."

Recently researchers in London analyzed nine randomized studies of aspirin users in the United States, Europe, and Japan. This study included 100,000 participants. These subjects had never had a heart attack or a stroke and took either an aspirin or a placebo. The goal was to see whether people would benefit from routinely taking an aspirin.

The data showed that those who took an aspirin regularly were 10 percent less likely than the others in the study to have any type of heart event and were 20 percent less likely to have a nonfatal heart attack. However, those who took an aspirin regularly were 30 percent more likely to develop serious gastrointestinal (GI) bleeding, which is a side effect of frequent aspirin use. The overall risk of dying for both aspirin users and nonusers was shown to be the same.

No anticancer benefit was found in this study. For every 162 people who took aspirin, the drug prevented one nonfatal heart attack but caused two serious bleeding events.*

Who should take aspirin? Among men who have had a heart attack, regular aspirin use lowers the risk of a second event by 20 to 30 percent. It also reduces the risk in women who have had a stroke caused by a blood clot.

In 2007, according to the US Agency for Healthcare Research and Quality, 19 percent of Americans regularly took aspirin. Among middle-aged aspirin users, the 2007 report found that 23 percent of

*Tara Parker-Pope, "Daily Aspirin Is Not for Everyone, Study Suggests," *New York Times* (January 16, 2012). Also available at http://well.blogs.nytimes.com/2012/01/16/daily-aspirin-is-not-for-everyone-study-suggests. Accessed September 26, 2012.

these aspirin users did not have established heart disease. Among older aspirin users, 41 percent did not have a history of stroke or heart attack.

Many people are taking this over-the-counter medication on their own without their doctor's knowledge. As the study described above confirms, there's serious risk of GI bleeding; and the number one cause of GI bleeding, which may lead to death, is the use of non-steroidal drugs. That's exactly what an aspirin is.

What's my advice? Research everything you put into your body, especially over-the-counter medications. Don't make assumptions. When it comes to my patients, if they have a strong history of heart disease or stroke or have experienced a cardiac event or stroke, I advise that they take an aspirin regularly. But I make absolutely sure there's no history or increased risk of bleeding.

I also advocate good hydration (drinking adequate water each day), exercise, and eating well to decrease other stressors that might put individuals at a higher risk. Drinking enough water helps thin the blood naturally. When the body is under stress, the blood wants to clot. So, whenever possible, stay away from excessively stressful situations, and keep your blood flowing freely.

+

facility—where more than half the patients are prescribed pain management narcotics for more than ninety days. Needless to say, this can be lucrative for the practitioner. My patient had a history of heart problems and also of cocaine use. At the time of the car accident, he'd been using cocaine for over a year. He was given narcotics for his pain. I doubt he was asked about other substances he was taking or counseled on the potential risks.

Two months ago, he suffered a fatal overdose of oxyco-done. His mother found him collapsed on the couch and rushed him to the hospital. His medical records revealed that in addition to the oxycodone and cocaine, he was taking an antidepressant prescribed by his psychiatrist. When I talked to his family, they expressed doubts that the forty-two-year-old would take any medications as prescribed. Rather he medicated himself as he saw fit. He misused drugs and paid a terrible price.

## Addictions

Many of the deaths resulting from the misuse of medications are related to addictions. In today's world we pursue passion that sometimes destroys the very essence of who we are and whom we love. We are putting enormous stress on our brains and bodies, stress that is damaging every organ system. We seek elaborate and often destructive ways to cope with the stress. In times gone by, we had the family unit to turn to. Now, however, the family unit is disintegrating right before our eyes.

An addiction to and misuse of medication may be an elaborate way to cope. Sometimes addictions develop because of the medications and their long-term effects on the brain. Many medications are considered addictive. Addiction is a complex topic, and much has been written on the subject. But for the purposes of this book, an addiction is a behavior pattern organized by frequent repetitions. It is a compulsive engagement in behavior that may have short-term rewards but in the end is destructive.

It is beyond the scope of this book to cover the topic of addictions in any detail, but some basics will help us understand the misuse of medication leading to deaths. Over time, addictive behaviors develop neural pathways in the brain. As these pathways are used, for whatever reason, in those addicted to medications, the pathways become very strong. As these pathways are used repetitively, the path becomes stronger and stronger. The first time, the pathway may be like a spider web. But as the behavior is repeated, the pathway becomes the equivalent of a string, and then a rope, and then a steel cable. The pathway can eventually be so strong that it affects behavior. Like a groove in a record, these pathways leading to behavior can be difficult to overcome because they are so automatic.

Let me give some examples. Complete the following items:

- Monday, Tuesday, _____
- 2, 4, 6, ____
- Good to the last _____
- I'd like to teach the world to _____.
- Mercury, Venus, Earth, _____

I think you get the picture. These pathways are interconnected to the entire brain and body. In addictions to medications, these pathways are extremely strong and have automatic triggers. More and more medication may be needed to satisfy the addictions. These addictions can be deadly if a pain medication, a medication affecting the brain or mood, is involved. This addictive behavior needs immediate attention. The final chapters of this book contain some suggestions to help if you or someone you know is having a problem with addictions and the misuse of medications.

## Legitimate Dangers

Many people do suffer from legitimate pain. As more and more painkilling medications are prescribed, the potential for abuse by doctors, pharmacists, patients, and criminals exists.

Let me toss out some statistics: according to the White House Office of National Drug Control Policy, "The annual milligram-per-person intake of opioids, such as oxycodone, increased from 74 milligrams to 369 milligrams from 1997–2007."[6] That's an increase of—get this—402 percent! Talk about the potential for misuse!

According to the National Institute on Drug Abuse, "an estimated 52 million people (20 percent of those aged 12 and older) have used prescription pain medications for *non-medical* reasons at least once in their lifetimes."[7] Regulations are increasing. This should help. The hope of these guidelines is that good doctors and pharmacists will catch patients who are shopping for lenient providers.

A study recently released by the *New England Journal of Medicine* reported that "116 million Americans battle pain of some sort on a daily basis, and doctors with a subspecialty in pain management believe chronic pain should be categorized as its own disease."[8]

Patients seek pain management for reasons from musculoskeletal pain to cancer. As a physician, it's hard for me to believe that all these prescriptions are legitimate. These medications can kill. They can stop the respiratory system cold. They can lead to mental impairments and interact with other medications, sometimes lethally. An article published in the *Journal of the American Medical Association* reported that in 2006 the death rate from overdose of prescription medications was 16.2 per 100,000.[9] If we extrapolate from that number, that would be 15,000 deaths per 300 million. The number of narcotics users has increased dramatically in the last six years. One West Virginia study concluded that opioid analgesics contributed to 93 percent of overdose deaths.[10]

As our world is becoming more stressed out than ever, people seek coping mechanisms to relieve the pain. Often they turn to medications, and an addiction can easily develop from there. Often these medications are unneeded and do not address the real problems behind the physical and mental discomfort. I've said it before and I'll say it again: the leading cause of death in America just might be medications. So, what is the real solution to our medication misuse problem? We'll look closer at this in later chapters.

# 6

# SLOW KILL AND DEADLY COMBINATIONS

*The least costly treatment for any illness is lethal medication.*
—WALTER E. DELLINGER

IF I WERE an evil person bent on destroying the human race, I wouldn't have to look far for a workable example of how to do that. First I'd make people sick in ways they didn't recognize. I'd get everyone happily eating health-destroying foods that tasted great but worked tirelessly in the background ingratiating themselves completely into the eater's brain. In other words, I'd get everyone addicted to harmful substances.

Is this happening today? Absolutely. I like the way Neal Barnard, MD, introduces this very danger in his book *Breaking the Food Seduction*: "You've felt the seduction. 'I know I shouldn't,' you tell yourself. But tastes and aromas call out like Sirens, leaving you little hope of resisting. We love food—and adore it sometimes—even when it doesn't love us back. Love is supposed to be nourishing and even invigorating, but sometimes our affairs with food pass from love to enslavement."[1]

We are also treating our minds in ways they were just not designed to be treated. Our brains were designed to be creative, not merely entertained. Our minds were designed to serve, not merely take. We were not designed to see murder, watch pornography, and live under constant stress. Computers, texting, tweeting, e-mailing—the constant information overload—are just a few of the many stressors changing the chemistry of the brain. There must be a balance. Constant stressors change our brains' chemistry, alter the ways we think and make decisions, and—you guessed it—cause us to look for coping mechanisms, some of which can cause additional damage.

So, here we are, "enslaved" by harmful foods and stressed-out brains that, in time, make us sick. And not just sick. They also make us fat and lazy and dull of mind. They rob us of our youth and spin our "sunset" years out of control, filling our days with doctor visits and an endless stream of—wait for it—medicines.

For many, trading the harmful effects of food and stress for the harmful effects of drugs is like jumping from the proverbial frying pan right into the fire. The destruction continues; only now it's not only the producers of seductive foods and the creators of all the information overload who are making fortunes off our eating habits, but the pharmaceutical companies that have begun raking in a large share of our hard-earned bucks.

Here's where that process gets totally ugly. Many drugs have the nasty habit of seducing us with pie-in-the-sky promises while slowly, over time, eroding our health potential. Like the food that got us here, we soon become tied to a medication with tight, painful bands. We're told that if we stop taking our pills, we'll die. Unfortunately, for many of us, if we *keep* taking our medications, we'll die. I call this phenomenon "slow kill."

## Deadly Blend

Not long ago, a strong, healthy, twenty-one-year-old football player from the University of Alabama died after attending a party in Florida. Blood tests administered after death revealed the presence of methadone (a narcotic), a muscle relaxant sold under the name Soma, diazepam (a tranquilizer commonly known as Valium), and trace amounts of oxycodone (a pain reliever) in his system. Each of these drugs carries hidden dangers. But when combined, they can produce the permanent side effect of death. This young man either didn't fully realize the terrible risks of mixing these medications, or he ignored them.[2]

A twenty-two-year-old linebacker from the University of Oklahoma died while visiting a friend. Toxicology reports revealed five prescription narcotics—oxymorphone, morphine, hydrocodone, hydromorphone, and oxycodone—in his bloodstream. He also was carrying a load of the tranquilizer alprazolam in his system. His death was deemed accidental.[3]

An article in the *New York Times* reported accidental overdosing from a wide variety of psychotropic medications. These are medications used to treat mental illnesses such as post-traumatic stress syndrome, depression, and anxiety. The autopsies revealed significant levels of the prescribed medication. These medications included antidepressants, antipsychotics, and sleep medications.[4] With mental health problems on the rise, there will be more deaths from respiratory and cardiovascular problems related to these medications. When people use these medications, side effects result, and—guess what—patients take an additional medication to help them cope, which compounds the problem.

While a particular drug may produce an adverse reaction with which you think you can live, combinations of drugs can create a real monster. Most prescription medications do not mix well with alcohol, cold medications, sleeping pills, antihistamines, pain relievers, and fever reducers. This can be a lethal mix. The problem is, people aren't educated about the long-term dangers of the drugs they dump down their throats. Access to these deadly doses is far too easy. Medications for pain, anxiety, and depression weren't designed for casual, I-don't-feel-well-today-so-I'll-just-pop-a-pill use. In our fast-paced, get-out-of-my-way world, pain—both physical and mental—is becoming as common as breathing. Our current mentality is to mask the symptoms while ignoring the causes.

This is generating a constant overuse of medications, and as a result, death rates are rising. People want to stop hurting, stop fearing, and stop worrying. Many are searching in the dark for help.

Think about it. When was the last time you saw a television commercial focusing solely on the *dangers* of a medication? At best you might hear the announcer say—usually in "rapid talk"—that there are some side effects and if you experience them, go see your doctor. Well, didn't you just do that? Why didn't he or she warn you about what you're going through?

Of course, there are no profits to be made if you *don't* take the medicine. Your getting well doesn't benefit anyone whose business it is to make you feel better.

---

## DID YOU KNOW?

Grapefruit juice interferes with liver enzymes needed to break down many medications: benzodiazepines, prescribed for anxiety; sertraline, used for depression; some statins used to lower cholesterol; verapamil, used for high blood pressure; the cough suppressant dextromethorphan; amiodarone, quinidine, disopyramide, and propafenone, used to treat rhythms; Viagra, used for impotence; codeine, oxycodone, and hydrocodone, used for pain; and zolpidem, used for insomnia. This is just a partial list. As you can surmise, if the liver cannot break down the medication, problems can arise, especially if many medications are being used at the same time. This is another possible example of how medications can slowly kill.

---

There's another element to medications about which few talk. Many drugs designed specifically for pain and anxiety not only deliver a degree of relief but also create a happy buzz. That's right. You really don't feel better. You just *think* you do. And, naturally, you want to continue to feel like that.

## Complex Interactions

It is estimated that 10 percent of the population drink alcohol daily and up to 70 percent consume alcohol occasionally. Consuming alcohol while taking certain medications that depress the central nervous system increases the sedative effects and impacts the ability to perform mental skills such as driving a car. Mixing alcohol with anti–Parkinson's disease drugs can lead to a dangerous increase in blood pressure, especially if a patient is already being treated for high blood pressure.

In people who regularly drink alcohol, certain important substances are depleted. One of these substances is called glutathione. This depletion damages the liver. Chronic alcohol ingestion also activates enzymes that metabolize acetaminophen, for example, into toxic by-products. This process can cause liver damage. This may sound complex, so let me simplify. When we take acetaminophen for pain or fever, our bodies have specific substances called enzymes that help break down the medication and eventually rid our bodies of it after it has accomplished the desired effect. Alcohol can change this process. It alters the mix of chemicals available to the liver, and the body can't get rid of the medication as it should. Extreme damage to the organs, in this case the liver, can occur.

The important point of all this is that interactions with medications are complex. Certain combinations of medications, when mixed with alcohol or pain medicines, can be fatal. Let's look at just two examples.

### Seldane

Seldane was marketed as the first medication for allergies that would not make users drowsy. Seldane alone did not pose much of a risk, but the potential for cardiac arrest developed. Seldane use was combined with the antibiotic erythromycin. The actual pharmaceutical effect was to change the electrical currents in the heart. An important interval called the QT interval was prolonged.

When Seldane was studied alone, no big problem. When combined with other medications that prolonged this interval in the heart's electrical system, the potential for a fatal heart rhythm developed. Seldane was on the market for twelve years before it was withdrawn because it was implicated in many deaths.

### Fen-Phen, the Deadly Duo

The combination of fenfluramine and phentermine was touted as a miracle drug to help in weight loss. Thousands flocked to this new medication with its promise of creating a new you through science. I'm grateful that I never prescribed it, but I sure gained a lot of patients after it was reported that it could damage heart valves. The FDA estimated that three to four million Americans had taken this medication for longer than three months. The frequency of heart valve damage was 22 percent for those who used it for shorter than three months. One-third of those who took the medication for longer than six months had serious heart valve damage.

Fenfluramine had been around for more than twenty years without serious problems. But the combination of fenfluramine and phentermine was proving deadly.

I can recall seeing patient after patient, asking how long each had been on the drug and ordering tests to evaluate their heart valves. I began to ask myself, *If this combo is deadly, how many other medications could have a similar effect when used together?*

## Chemical Reactions

It's naive to think that anyone can predict how an outside chemical will react inside the body. When you add several more chemicals, coupled with underlying medical conditions that can diminish and change how the body metabolizes medications, you have the potential for disaster.

Keep in mind that medications are usually studied in healthy patients and not in combination with other drugs or in very sick patients. Unfortunately, that particular part of the "study" is left to consumers. Most of my patients suffer from more than one illness and seek treatment from more than one doctor. One of my current patients is seeing an internist, a cardiologist, a pulmonologist, a nephrologist, a gastroenterologist, a neurologist, and an orthopedic surgeon. This patient is taking nearly twenty medications. She, unfortunately, is not alone in that.

As time goes by, and as newer and more potent drugs are introduced into mainstream medicine, scientists are discovering that these drugs can slowly, methodically, damage the body, including the brain. It is impossible to understand with any degree of certainty how these medications will interact with other medications, accompanying illnesses, and aging organs.

We know certain medications raise the risk of heart attack. Others increase the chance of suicide. Some increase the risk of bleeding, while still others may elicit fatal heart rhythms. There are also those that set the stage for anaphylaxis. These are all *known* adverse reactions.

What we don't know is *how* these medications work when combined. So, in the short run, we must force ourselves to weigh the inherent risks against the benefits. If the benefits are limited and the risks could be life threatening, we must think twice. However, this is often impossible to know when we don't understand the full ramifications of taking these medications. This leaves us—physicians and patients—scratching our collective heads and wondering which is worse: the condition or the treatment? The ill or the pill?

## Breakdown Products

Many medications are broken down in the liver by a process called the p450 enzyme system. When numerous medications are passed through this system, it becomes overwhelmed, and each drug—which was originally studied using a normal, not overwhelmed, p450 enzyme system—becomes a cog in a spinning, out-of-control wheel. The liver simply can't handle all the medications waiting to be processed, and some of the "breakdown products"—the result of this synthesis—become toxic to the body. These toxins travel to various parts of the human anatomy and wait for an opportune time to begin their poisonous work. Slow kill.

Years ago, the medication Posicor hit the shelves. This drug utilized the body's internal p450 system, and because of this, the product label warned against using Posicor with at least twenty-five other medications—drugs that also utilize the p450 system. In spite of the warning, many patients were experiencing dangerously slow heart rates and other adverse reactions. In our multidrug society, Posicor had become dangerous. In June of 1999, it was quietly withdrawn from the market.

The truth is, we really don't know how all these medications are reacting and whether or not the products of the partially broken-down drug will cause a serious problem down the road. As I've said before, we become test cases for the drug companies.

Think about this: it is estimated that at least three billion prescriptions are written in the United States each year. This does not include our use of over-the-counter medications, unregulated herbs, and various nutritional supplements. We've got an industry without adequate safeguards where profit is often king, a society wanting a quick fix, and a system that turns its head the other way when something bad happens. Medicines can kill, and we're allowing it to happen.

## Performance Enhancement

Whether we're at work or at home, we all want to enhance our performance. In recent years we have seen numerous stories about the use of performance-enhancing substances. I call these performance-enhancing *medications*. Cyclist Lance Armstrong has been accused of using them. Before being acquitted of perjury charges, pitcher Roger Clemens went through a long, drawn-out court battle related to his testimony before Congress concerning use of these medications. José Canseco and Barry Bonds have been accused. Students use stimulants to keep them studying longer. Baseball players, cyclists, Olympians, wrestlers, body builders, and youth wanting to be "buff" have been implicated. An entire generation is experimenting with the off-label use of these performance-enhancing medications. What are the implications?

Thyroid medications, steroids, testosterone, growth factors such as hCG, stimulants such as methamphetamines, and other substances have all been mentioned as performance enhancers. These might improve short-term performance, but what are they doing over the long haul?

Some time ago a story of a wrestler who died of "roid rage" hit the papers. Long-term steroid use causes a host of potentially fatal problems, including infections from a weakened immune system, problems with the adrenal gland, and a condition called osteonecrosis that affects the bones. The changes in behavior are startling. Testosterone can stimulate cancer growth. Stimulants can trigger life-threatening abnormal heart rhythms. These medications have specific medical usages. Are they killing in ways unperceivable at this time? I suspect the answer is yes. We might have to wait years to evaluate the effects. Those who use performance-enhancing drugs would prefer a short-term reward and take a chance in the future. After all, modern medicine can "fix" the problem.

✛

### THE UNBORN

You may have children or grandchildren or you may hope to have children someday. My children, Kelli and Jake, light up my life. Unfortunately, medications have killed and are killing the unborn. When a person is developing in the womb, many medications can do harm. We call a medication that harms in this manner a *teratogen*. This comes from a Greek word meaning "monster forming" (an unfortunate term that goes back to ancient superstitions that saw any plant or animal or human with a deformity as a reflection of an omen, or warning, of something negative). The phrase has lost its original meaning over the centuries, and I want to make it abundantly clear that we do not consider these precious babies monsters in any way. The first teratogen I was introduced to in medical school was the drug thalidomide. I can remember seeing the pictures of the deformed bodies of these children whose mothers had used the medication while pregnant. Those photos made a lasting impression on me.

Birth defects are the leading cause of infant mortality in the United States, accounting for 20 percent of the deaths. Three to 5 percent of newborns have some type of birth defect. In other words, in one thousand births, statistically we can expect to see thirty to fifty of those babies with birth defects. Teratogenic medications have been implicated both in birth defects and in subsequent deaths. Lithium carbonate, used to treat some psychiatric disorders; the blood thinner warfarin; the class of blood pressure medications called ACE inhibitors; tretinoin for the skin; anticancer medications; antithyroid medications; Accutane for acne; Dilantin for seizures; methotrexate for psoriasis; and tetracycline for bacterial infections are just a few of the teratogens available for use. In addition, antidepressants can increase the overall risk of miscarriage.

Every time I see a woman of childbearing age, I wonder whether she is taking a medication that could potentially harm an unborn child. Then I wonder whether there is sufficient information available about some of the medications being prescribed—especially those newer to the market—to determine the hidden effects of these medications on the unborn. No one would ever have released the morning sickness medication thalidomide if there had been knowledge about its potential to cause severe birth defects. Over the course of one long-term scientific study, a group of 488,175 women ages fourteen to forty-four received a total of more than one million prescription medications. One in six of these women received a medication that could cause a birth defect. This study concluded that the women were no more likely to receive special counseling about the danger of birth defects than those receiving less-risky medications.[1]

Another growing problem is the skyrocketing drug abuse by pregnant women who are passing their addictions on to their unborn babies. A University of Michigan report shows that between 2000

---

[1] Eleanor Bimla Schwarz et al, "Documentation of Contraception and Pregnancy When Prescribing Potentially Teratogenic Medications for Reproductive-Age Women," *Annals of Internal Medicine* 147 (2007): 370–76.

and 2009, the number of infants born addicted to opiates such as Oxycontin and Vicodin tripled to more than 13,500 per year, or about one birth an hour. In the same period, the number of women using opiates increased fivefold.[2] Babies born to these women suffer from prematurity, are underweight, and can suffer from withdrawal in their early weeks as newborns. With an estimated 16 percent of teens and 8 percent of pregnant women between 18 and 25 using illicit drugs, the unborn are at serious risk from these drugs that can potentially kill.

We also need to mention the drug mifepristone, more commonly known as RU-486. This drug was developed in France to terminate intrauterine pregnancies. No matter when you believe life begins, the heart has already begun beating by around three and a half weeks after conception. This medication ends the pregnancy and also has the potential to cause dangerous bleeding in the mother.

I have never seen a yearly mortality figure on how many of the unborn die as a result of a birth defect, but I am sure it is not zero. And I suspect the number of medical abortions from RU-486 is rising worldwide.

---

[2]Genevra Pittman, "More US Babies Born to Mothers Who Abuse Painkillers," *Chicago Tribune* (May 1, 2012). Also available at http://articles.chicagotribune.com/2012-05-01/news/sns-rt-usa-addictionnewbornsl4e8g 17jm-20120501_1_opiates-maternal-drug-abuse-babies. Accessed October 5, 2012.

---

✦

## Number One

As I have stated earlier, I believe medications are the number one cause of death in America. The data is hard to come by, but I believe the common sense to make this statement is not. Let me review some facts once again to emphasize this point.

In 2003 Gary Null, PhD, wrote the article "Death by Medicine," in which he estimates that 106,000 deaths from in-hospital adverse drug reactions, 98,000 from medical errors, and 199,000 from outpatient drug reactions take place yearly. That's 400,000 lives snuffed out from what's supposed to cure them of their illnesses. This was a landmark report because medical professionals simply did not report the bad results, although many of us working in the trenches suspected the problem.

Dr. Lucien Leape's 1997 medical and drug error rate of three million (that means three million total errors for the prescriptions written) multiplied by the fatality rate of 14 percent gives an annual death rate—just from errors—of 420,000. Remember, Dr. Leape's findings were published more than ten years ago. Since that time, the numbers of prescription medications, as well as access to over-the-counter medications, have skyrocketed. Three billion plus prescriptions dramatically increase the error rate today as compared to the error rate used back in 1997. If Dr. Leape's data were used with the number of prescriptions written today, the numbers would be astounding. To these numbers add deaths from the narcotics epidemic, deaths from anaphylaxis and adverse reactions, deaths from patient mistakes, deaths from rising mental health problems and the drugs prescribed to combat mental illness (this problem and the medications used to treat it are at epidemic proportions), deaths from misuse of medications, and deaths from the obesity epidemic and the subsequent prescriptions written for the myriad of obesity-related problems. Common sense indicates that the number one cause of death in America is not cardiovascular disease. Medications are the number one cause of death.

In 2007 the Centers for Disease Control (CDC) reported approximately 616,000 deaths from cardiovascular disease, 567,000 from cancer, and 135,000 from strokes.[5]

Where is the number related to deaths from medications? We'll probably never know. Why? Because mistakes by medical personnel, manufacturers, and patients; adverse reactions; accidents caused by medications; overdosages; and underappreciated damage from these medications simply aren't reported in full. It only makes sense that as more and more medications are prescribed and as more and more over-the-counter drugs find their way into our medicine cabinets, these numbers will continue to rise. We also don't have to be rocket scientists to figure out that the 420,000 figure mentioned above is probably a very, very conservative number.

I am a cardiologist. I try to prevent deaths from cardiovascular disease. But I can't help but conclude—after studying the preceding numbers—that my time might be better spent combating deaths from medicine and educating the world about the dangers of taking prescription drugs than seeing patients. I might save more lives in the long run!

Countless books have been written about the leading causes of death. Daily research is done to combat these terrible illnesses. The media focuses on these issues. Yet there is a scarcity of books and articles on the fact that medicines are killing us. Why don't we have a "Worldwide Society for the Prevention of Death by Medications"? Why aren't there reams of material reflecting accurate reporting and research along with widespread media coverage on this subject?

## A Medicated Zombie

Mr. Williams was brought to see me so I could check his heart. He was failing to thrive, couldn't think correctly, and was basically what his family described as a "zombie."

None of the tests on his heart showed any obvious problems. But as I explored Mr. Williams's medical history, I discovered that in his forties he began taking a medication for blood pressure, which had been prescribed after just one blood pressure reading in his doctor's office.

Five years later, he began taking a diabetes medication. Still later, he received a medication to help him sleep. One doctor thought he was depressed, and an antidepressant joined the other little pills in his medicine cabinet. But his slow journey to my office was just beginning.

When he began complaining of pain, his doctor prescribed an anti-inflammatory medicine. When this did not help, a pain specialist prescribed a narcotic. Because Mr. Williams moved little, he started to retain fluids, and a diuretic and a potassium replacement were added.

His thyroid was a little off, so a thyroid medication joined the others. He didn't eat well, so an appetite stimulant and an antacid were prescribed by a gastroenterology specialist.

When he seemed to lack interest in life, he saw a psychiatrist, who added another antidepressant, as well as a memory pill in the hope of helping combat his forgetfulness. Mr. Williams moved from doctor to doctor, and always left his appointments with a brand-new prescription tucked in his jacket pocket.

He finally reached the stage where he needed a lot of care, and he moved in with his family in a new town. They wanted to put him in hospice because, at age sixty-eight, he was dying. Yes, he was dying, not from a disease but from all the medications he was taking.

When those pills and potions were carefully withdrawn, Mr. Williams got better—a lot better. The last time he came to see me, he told me he was having a blast playing with his grandchildren. That's a long way from hospice!

I see this same situation to some degree every day. As I evaluate patients in nursing homes and look at the long lists of medications those precious people are taking, I wonder how many really need everything that has been prescribed. How many are experiencing the slow kill that comes as a result of both the blending of pharmaceuticals and the years those medications have had access to the human body?

### Antibiotics

How are antibiotics slowly killing? It has been estimated that over three million pounds of antibiotics are used each year on humans. A few years ago the population in America was 284 million. This would equate to 10 teaspoons of pure antibiotics a year for each person.[6] In 2003, the CDC cited tens of millions of unnecessary antibiotic prescriptions written for viral infections.[7] An amazing 50 percent of patients with upper respiratory infections receive antibiotics from their doctors.[8] The CDC estimates that 90 percent of upper respiratory infections are viral and should not be treated with an antibiotic.[9] In a pediatric study, prescriptions for antibiotics were shown to be written 62 percent of the time if the parents expected an antibiotic and 7 percent of the time if parents did not.[10] Another study showed that antibiotics were written for upper respiratory infections 68 percent of the time.[11] Eighty percent of those prescriptions were not needed. More than a billion dollars were spent on antibiotics inappropriately prescribed for adult upper respiratory infections.[12] These are just a few of the many studies that leave no doubt: antibiotics are overused.

Using antibiotics when they are not needed can lead to the development of deadly strains of bacteria that are resistant to drugs. Deadly strains of bacteria that are resistant to drugs caused more than 88,000 deaths due to hospital-acquired infections.[13] This is especially a problem in hospitals where infections are occurring and sometimes being spread from patient to patient. When you really need an antibiotic, your infection may be resistant to it.

When we are finished with an antibiotic or any other prescription medicine, how do we typically dispose of the waste? Where do the breakdown products of the antibiotics and other prescriptions and over-the-counter medications go? With tons of medications used in all aspects of life, this is a legitimate question and concern. Most of the medication, both the unused medication and the breakdown products we eliminate, is flushed down the toilet. These substances end up in our water supply. The water treatment centers cannot take care of all the medications and breakdown products hitting the system. We have no idea what the long-term effects are. Slow kill, perhaps? One thing I can say for sure is that this is not making us healthier.

## Mind over Matter

John stopped by my office one sunny afternoon and told me he had been in a car accident some time ago. No alcohol was involved, but the man who plowed into John's car was a diabetic and had numerous documented episodes of low blood sugar—a condition that caused him to pass out. That makes me wonder once again how many accidents, crimes, and drownings might have been prevented if people on medications had been able to think clearly. They may have been on their medications for years. "The pills don't cause me any problems," they'd say. Then one day they find themselves sitting in a twisted pile of metal, or standing over a gunshot victim, or unable to fight the rush of water entering their lungs.

Methamphetamine, a chemical substance similar to pseudoephedrine, found in over-the-counter medications, speeds up the metabolism.

A sheriff's deputy pulled over a pregnant nineteen-year-old Georgia woman, her boyfriend, and her mother during a traffic stop. The young woman suddenly began acting irrationally. It was later discovered that she was hiding a bag of meth in her vagina. Later interviews revealed that she'd told her mom and boyfriend just before the incident,

"Give the meth to me; I'll hide it. No one will search me because I'm pregnant." But the contents of the bag seeped into her body, poisoning her and her unborn child. The baby was delivered stillborn a day before its young mother passed away.

What a tragic story! Yet many are taking medications, chemicals, and mixtures that could lead to the same result. These medications often affect the mind, transforming a perfectly rational being into someone who thinks illogically . . . and acts illogically. The side effect of altered thinking and the inability to reason rationally doesn't show up in medical statistics unless, as in this case, someone is there to recognize the changes and start an investigation.

## An Adverse Reaction to High Heels

Before we come to the end of this chapter focusing on how medicines kill over time, I want to relate the following story. Being someone who spends his days (and a lot of his nights) trying to lead people from where they are to where they want to be requires more than following the status quo. It demands that I step back and look at the big picture while also keeping one eye on the trends. It also requires honesty and truth. Sometimes the truth hurts.

Some time ago a pleasant, middle-aged woman came to me complaining of chest pains. Her story is interesting and bears repeating. She'd been an executive assistant at an important business office. The standard of dress of her company required that the women there wear high-heeled shoes. This she did faithfully.

However, after years of cramming her feet into these shoes, she needed to see a podiatrist because of severe foot pain. After two operations, she was still unable to walk comfortably—thus causing her to become inactive. The inability to walk and exercise brought on weight gain, which caused her to develop diabetes, hypertension (high blood pressure), and sleep apnea and to take numerous medications, which were supposed to ease her many symptoms.

Her world was falling apart. She required a sleep mask at night and, because of her suffering, began taking narcotics and sleeping pills. Her missed days at work, deepening health issues, and inability to think clearly contributed to her losing her job. But that wasn't all.

The narcotics slowed her bowels and further diminished her ability to think clearly. She was placed on more powerful sleeping pills and a medication for depression. Unfortunately, she developed a small bowel obstruction, which was complicated by infection. That's when the chest pains began.

Isolated story? Hardly. I see variations of this theme each and every day as I make my rounds in the hospital. I talk to people on our radio shows and hear from viewers of my television programs. This story is incredibly common.

If it's not high heels, it's job stress, small injuries, bad eating habits, tight-fitting clothes, environmental issues, busy schedules, misinformation, dangerous traditions—the list goes on and on. All begin innocently enough. All set in motion the slow kill that medications bring into the mix.

If we could go back to the start of the problem, if we would just ask the question *why* and concentrate on finding the answer to that question, many problems with medications could be avoided completely.

I may be criticized severely for saying what I say. But one of the promises I made when I became a doctor was to "do no harm." Medicines can kill quickly or slowly. They can change the way we think and feel. Even the drugs I depend on in my own field of healing can indirectly take over the lives of my patients. I don't like that! That "takeover" may not be as obvious to others as the dark lines on the arms of the heroin addict or the slurred speech and uninhibited actions of the alcoholic, but something is happening, something lethal.

It's time to stop the slow kill and begin the healing. We will cover the solutions in a just few chapters, but here's a sneak preview: true healing comes from following the laws of health set in place long ago in a Garden formed by the hand of a loving Creator—the same Creator who made the people he designed, literally from the ground up, to live there. It's there that we find the answers to today's health crises. It's there we'll find the answer to the question why. It's there we'll uncover the most powerful medications this world will ever know.

# 7

# OVER-THE-COUNTER MEDICATIONS

*He who lives by medical prescription lives miserably.*
—LATIN PROVERB

OVER-THE-COUNTER (OTC) medications may be sold and consumed without a prescription. Anyone can purchase these substances at a variety of places, from drugstores to supermarkets to even the local gas station. The OTC drugs treat symptoms, whether stuffiness from a cold, a tension headache, acid reflux, or drowsiness. These drugs are popular because they help consumers save money and time by not needing to see a health care provider. They are usually very well marketed to all ages.

In fact, OTC medications are a growing market. According to the Nielsen Company, retail sales of OTCs in the US in 2010 (excluding sales by Walmart) were worth $17 billion.[1]

This is a $3 billion increase over a ten-year period. In 2001, the FDA reported more than eighty classes of OTC medications. According to the 2011 report of the Consumer Healthcare Products Association (CHPA), "there are approximately 1,000 active ingredients used in the more than 100,000 OTC products available in the marketplace today."[2] Today OTC drugs contain ingredients that were available only by prescription in the past. Most of us use these OTC medications. However, there can be problems. The active ingredients can be deadly. An example of one of these is ephedrine.

## Ephedrine

Some time ago, two brothers, ages five and two, died of hyperthermia (extremely high body temperature). One was brought to the hospital lifeless, and despite everything medicine could offer, this innocent child died. They were reportedly left unattended in a car, where temperatures reached a searing 120 degrees. Their mother was nowhere to be found. She later faced murder and methamphetamine charges. According to police, the evidence showed that the mother actually made the meth that played a role in their deaths. She was not taking care of her children. The active ingredient in meth is ephedrine. But this ingredient is also present in many OTC medications.

Chemically, ephedrine has a similar structure to amphetamine and methamphetamine. The Chinese stimulant ma huang contains ephedrine. This substance has been around a long time. It is used in many OTC cold medications to help dilate the bronchial tubes and relieve congestion. It is also used to make methamphetamines ("speed"). Ephedrine is an active ingredient in many OTC weight-loss products because it "speeds up" the metabolism. The death of Baltimore Orioles pitcher Steve Bechler was attributed to ephedrine he was using as a weight-loss medication and energy booster.[3] Back in 1998, researchers linked ephedrine to at least seventeen deaths.[4] This OTC active ingredient can kill, and yet it is readily available.

Ephedrine causes an increase in blood pressure. Fashion designer Anne Marie Capati took ephedrine as a fat burner. She collapsed and died from a stroke, an uncontrollable bleeding in her brain. Capati had preexisting high blood pressure. She was only thirty-seven.[5] Ephedrine can also cause dangerous heart rhythms, heart attack, stroke, confusion, hallucinations, hostility, panic, and shortness of breath, to name just a few of its side effects. In people who are dehydrated, who have high blood pressure or congenital heart disease, and who take certain antidepressant medications, ephedrine could be lethal. As society looks to lose weight quickly, have more energy, or treat cold symptoms, the use of ephedrine will increase. It's likely the number of fatalities will too. No one knows how many.

### Impotence

No man likes this word. Yet it has been estimated that thirty million men suffer from ED, or erectile dysfunction. The blockbuster medicine sildenafil, sold under the name Viagra, was a help, but if those who used it were also taking nitroglycerin products in the treatment of cardiovascular disease, the result could be fatally low blood pressure. Many men with cardiovascular disease use nitroglycerin and also have ED. They come to me, and I warn them of the dangers. Then they look for other solutions. They go the OTC route. And guess what? There are many herbal supplements that promise help. Unfortunately, their ingredients have the same lethal potential when mixed with nitroglycerin products. Taking OTC medications has risks.

## Phenylpropanolamine/PPA

In past years PPA was used in more than four hundred OTC medications. Most of these have been used to treat symptoms associated with the common cold, which is rarely deadly, and in weight-loss medications. A study from Yale University showed an increased risk of hemorrhagic stroke (bleeding in the brain) in those who used OTCs containing PPA.[6] This substance was banned in November 2000 in the States but is still available in Europe. When this was banned, a similar substance to achieve similar results was needed. You guessed it: ephedrine, a similar compound, was introduced. PPA was around for sixty years before something was done. How many lives were lost? Was the problem of dangerous ingredients in OTC medications solved?

## Dextromethorphan

Dextromethorphan is an active ingredient found in many OTC cough suppressants. No one likes to cough. However, many are using this ingredient to get high. On the street it is known by many names, including Candy, Rojo, Skittles, or just by its brand name, Robitussin. The *Journal of the Annals of Toxicology* reported five deaths of teenagers who were using dextromethorphan "recreationally." Most of the reported deaths have been from overdoses.[7] The CDC estimated in 2004–2005 that 1,519 children ages two and younger were treated in emergency departments for adverse reactions related to cold medications.[8] Some did not survive.

## Acetaminophen

Acetaminophen, known more commonly by its brand name, Tylenol, is probably the most-used pain reliever in the world, but this ingredient, which is available to all, can cause death. In June 2003, Kellie McWilliams was suffering from a migraine. She took acetaminophen, reportedly twenty of the 500 mg capsules, trying to get relief. The maximum recommended dose is no more than 3,000 mg in twenty-four hours. Kellie became ill with kidney and liver damage that resulted in organ failure.[9] An article in the journal *Hepatology* revealed that the most common cause of acute liver failure is acetaminophen.[10] Even though this is rare, one must be careful with any OTC medication.

I could go on and on about how OTC medications can

+

## TIPS FOR SAFE OTC MEDICATION USE

- Read the warnings.
- Look for the active ingredients and learn about them.
- Know which of your medications might interact with OTC medications.
- Know what medical conditions might affect the use of OTC medications.
- Take the correct dose listed on the package insert.
- Talk to your pharmacist, doctor, or other provider about OTC medications.
- If your symptoms are minimal, do not take an OTC medication.
- If your symptoms worsen or do not go away, seek a professional's advice.
- Let your health care provider know of OTC medications you take on a regular basis, including these potentially dangerous common herbs:

  1. Ephedrine speeds up the metabolism and can increase the risk of abnormal heart rhythms. (See the discussion on pages 119–120.)
  2. Licorice root works as a diuretic, causing a loss of potassium.
  3. Ginkgo biloba thins the blood. Be careful if you are taking prescription blood thinners.
  4. St. John's wort may alter the effectiveness of antidepressants.
  5. Valerian and kava kava are sedatives.
  6. Digitalis is dangerous if you take medications that slow the heart or if you have kidney failure.
  7. Celery seed, horsetail, and dandelion leaf are natural diuretics and can throw electrolytes off balance.
  8. Foxglove can produce dangerous heart rhythms.
  9. Wormwood is a central nervous system depressant.
  10. Yohimbine can lower blood pressure.

To learn more, consult the *Physicians' Desk Reference for Herbal Medicines* or visit www.nlm.nih.gov/medlineplus/herbalmedicine.html.

+

kill. Sometimes the symptoms of a cold or other illness that is rarely life threatening are less a risk than taking an OTC. Rarely do I find people who actually read the labels to learn about the OTC and the herbs they are ingesting. When mixed with medical conditions such as hypertension or dehydration, these OTC medications pose a greater risk than usual. In the very young, the active ingredients in OTCs, as we have noted, can be very dangerous and sometimes lethal. Yes, OTCs, like prescription medications, have the potential to kill. Since the OTCs are not prescribed, there is less supervision over how they are used. When users are already taking certain other medications, the risks can similarly skyrocket. We are now becoming increasingly aware of the dangers. If we are going to self-medicate, we must be wise.

IN PART 1, I explained my belief that medications are the number one cause of death. I have presented what I firmly believe is a logical argument for that belief in the light of common sense, personal experience as a physician trained in modern medicine, and the limited availability of statistics. Remember, complete statistical data simply does not exist, nor do I expect, in this day, to find such data, the existence of which would simply not be politically correct.

To review briefly, we have looked at how medicines kill both in the hospital and in the outpatient world. I have demonstrated how medication mistakes are made at all levels, from production to labeling to dispersing to prescribing. I have told stories of how mistakes are made by providers as well as by patients. We've looked at deaths from anaphylaxis as well as fatalities from other adverse reactions. Sometimes these adverse reactions were a known risk; other times no one discovered the risks until a medication had been on the market for a while. We've talked about the misuse of medications, the growing problem that misuse represents, and the many aspects of how medications might be slowly killing our organs, including our brains. Whenever possible I've used the available statistics to support my statements.

The stories you read in part 1 are true. I would not be writing this book if I had not seen them and believed, with all my heart, in the need to make others aware of the problem. However, awareness is not enough. Something more is needed. Unfortunately I do not expect a government grant or pharmaceutical funding to help. It will be up to you, as you read this, to take the next step. But before any of us take the next step, let me tell you about a doctor I know.

This doctor had been trained by the best medical mentors in the land. Hours and hours of study, many hours treating countless patients with all types of problems, and then years of clinical practice were all part of his ongoing training, and yet something seemed to be missing. One day he found a physician who changed his entire concept of medicine. Let me explain.

In the 1800s, if doctors did not use leeches to pull blood from patients with fevers, they were considered "bad" doctors. In the 1930s, physicians prescribed smoking ciga-rettes to treat patients with asthma.

Medicine had also made some major advancements throughout history. There was the invention of anesthesia. This opened the field of modern surgery. Now diseased gall-bladders and appendixes could be removed. Bowels could be repaired. Bleeding could be stopped, and a host of prob-lems could be "fixed." We could now address the problem of patients dying from the pain and the physical shock of surgery.

Antibiotics were discovered. Infections that had once killed now had a treatment. Along came vaccines, which helped eradicate more disease. Hearts that would have stopped were now kept going by pacemakers. Defibrillators restored or maintained heart rhythms in dangerous situa-tions. Stents and powerful medicines were developed to treat heart attacks. Technology was also able to peer deep inside the body and find out what was wrong. Unfortunately, as technology in general advanced, more problems developed. Dr. Joel J. Nobel noted, "The purpose of medicine is to pre-vent significant disease, to decrease pain and to postpone death. Technology has to support these goals; if not, it may be counterproductive."[1]

Lifestyle diseases were becoming more and more of a problem. The substances we put into our bodies and minds were causing problems. We were gaining weight, developing stressed-out minds, and putting a new set of chemicals in our bodies, and more and more medications were developed to deal with the plethora of symptoms.

This is the setting in which the doctor I am talking about was trained. The professional literature and training clearly demonstrated that modern medicine had an important place. And yet, new problems were developing in the masses. Simple logic made this doctor realize that medicine was heading down a dangerous path. There was certainly a need for modern medicine, especially for acute problems, but the problems of excess were not being handled in the best way. Medicines were easy to take and were a quick fix, but were the negative effects worth the risks? Was modern medicine addressing the underlying causes of the symptoms? The doctor looked back over the centuries and saw the great healers of all time giving advice, beginning with Hippocrates: "First, do no harm." Throughout the course of history there were warnings about too much medicine. Were we heeding these warnings? Was modern medicine now out of control? Were the patients' demands driving the system or were the profit margins? As this doctor looked at the history of medicine and at where modern medicine was going, he wondered, *In another one hundred years, how will the future judge today's practice of medicine?*

This doctor began a quest for answers outside his training. He knew this could be a slippery slope, but he plunged onward. He needed a new mentor to guide him and to give him the courage to go against the tide. That's when he found the Great Physician. This Physician was able to heal physical disease by miracles. He could also heal the soul. It was time to embrace a new set of ideas. This Physician-Healer had given a Manual that applied to medicine as well as to life. Would that Manual throw out the good in modern medicine and technology? Absolutely not! But there needed to be a balance between the two, and the scales were being tipped.

If you haven't already guessed, I was this doctor. But I was becoming someone different—or, perhaps, more—than what I was trained to be in medical school, internal medicine residency, cardiology fellowship, and the years in clinical practice. My training was excellent and needed. But now my eyes were being opened to the problems you've been reading about. I knew that talking about the problems was not enough. I had to try to give each one of you reading this book some ways to find solutions and to avoid the problems we've been discussing.

We live in an imperfect world, and I am learning the importance of loving and not judging. Changing a system starts with one person at a time making little changes, one at a time. One change leads to another. To change a system, we must realize that the system needs to change. As you have surmised, one of the changes needed is a decrease in the use of medications. That decrease would mean fewer deaths from medications. The benefit seems obvious. As we move into part 2, I will offer some possible solutions to our overmedicated world.

# 8

# SOMETIMES YOU NEED TO THINK

*When you treat a disease, first treat the mind.*
**—CHEN JEN**

ACCORDING TO THE Centers for Disease Control, over the last ten years the percentage of Americans who took at least one prescription drug in the past month increased from 44 percent to 48 percent. The use of two or more drugs increased from 25 percent to 31 percent, and the use of five or more drugs increased from 6 percent to 11 percent. In 2007 and 2008, one in five children and nine of ten older Americans reported using at least one prescription medication in the preceding month. In 2008, spending on prescription drugs, not including over-the-counter medications, was $234 billion, which was double what was spent in 1999.[1] These trends continue in 2013. We must think carefully before we take a medication: Is the risk worth the benefit? And are there other options to consider?

## Jenna

Jenna was the ideal patient. She did not want to take medications unnecessarily. Through the years we had been able to change her chemistry in other ways. She was eating better, exercising, and resting enough, but she was discouraged because she was still taking two medications. As we sat and talked, I explained that health is partly determined by the food we eat and also by our hydration, rest, body weight, and activity level. There is also a genetic component, and to complicate matters, there are factors in our lives that can activate both good genetics and bad genetics.

When Dr. Francis Collins's team on the Human Genome Project finished sequencing the human genome, or genetic material, we began to have not only more tools to understand science and medicine but also a greater understanding of the complexity we're dealing with. For example, we've known for some time that cigarette use has been associated with cancer. Getting too much sun, to the point of burning, has been associated with skin cancer. Exposure to certain substances in our environment, such as asbestos, can trigger cancer.

Now science is realizing that many other factors alter the way our body chemistry is regulated. We are learning that obesity can affect how our bodies make certain proteins. These days, most people are familiar with the term *DNA*, which refers to the genetic material that determines who we are. Segments of DNA are called genes. Various factors, including obesity, can regulate this genetic material and affect how the genes manage the body's chemistry. It goes without saying that the way the genes express themselves is very complex. Gene expression, as well as our overall genetic makeup, definitely plays a role in our health.

## Joseph

Joseph, fifty-eight, came to my office after having surgery to open his right coronary artery. He exercised daily, ate a near-perfect diet, never smoked, was not a diabetic, and had perfect blood pressure and cholesterol levels. His first question to me was, "How could I have had a heart attack?"

I answered, "How old was your dad when he had his first heart problem?"

"Thirty-four," Joseph replied.

"Then," I said, "I guess your healthy living has made a positive difference."

The point I was trying to make to Joseph and to Jenna, as well as to you, is that there are things over which we just do not have control. We did not choose our moms and dads. Having a parent with cardiovascular disease, as Joseph did, may mean that we are more prone to develop the same problem ourselves. Joseph was doing everything right, and that improved his health significantly, but it could not eliminate a genetic predisposition to heart disease that he inherited from his father. At this time in history, we are learning more and more about how certain aspects of our genes can affect our health, and yes, sometimes we need to take a medication. Sometimes the risk is worth it. But each time, we need to ask the more important question: *Is the risk involved in taking this medicine worth the benefit we will gain from it?*

I have this discussion with people taking blood thinners (also known as anticoagulants) regularly. Sure, taking an aspirin regularly has a small chance of causing stomach bleeding. And yes, given the right set of circumstances, there is a small chance of bleeding to death, but it is an extremely small chance. Other blood thinners I prescribe, including warfarin (sometimes sold under the name Coumadin), are more potent against clots but also significantly increase the risk of bleeding.

As I had this discussion with Jenna about the possibility that she might have to remain on these medications and that perhaps the risks were worth it, she asked, "Is there anything else that might be playing a role?"

I thought for a moment and said, "Yes. Your brain and thought processes could be playing a role." I explained to her that the way we think plays a role in our health. This is more involved than just making choices about the risks and benefits of a medication.

Mrs. Smith came to the office on a Friday afternoon. I enjoy Friday afternoons because I have a little more time to talk with my patients. Ten minutes with an established patient and twenty minutes with a new one do not seem to be enough time for me. Fridays are a little bit more relaxed. When Mrs. Smith came for her appointment, she explained how she came to be my patient. My first question to her was, "Mrs. Smith, why did you have a heart attack?" She did not know, nor had she given this any thought. But eventually she began asking me questions: "Why am I on this medication?" "Is it possible to be off this medication?" She was beginning to think more deeply about her health.

I often see patients who just accept the status quo, never ask why, never actually think for themselves. Unfortunately, they are the majority. If my doctor or someone on television or the Internet or whoever tells me something, it must be true, right? Who are we to question? I want Jenna and all my other patients, as well as you, to realize that the brain plays a major role in our health and genetics. Not only is it important to have a healthy brain to make decisions and ask the *why* questions, but the brain regulates the entire body, and a healthy brain can help keep us away from dangerous medications.

My colleague and friend Dr. Tim Jennings, a psychiatrist and president of the Tennessee Psychiatric Association, has opened my eyes to the importance of the brain in maintaining physical health. Ordinarily cardiologists and psychiatrists do not usually interact much, but I believe that God brought him into my life to open my eyes to the importance of the brain. In my practice I had not really thought much about my patients' brains. I was focused on their hearts and on nutrition, healthy lifestyles, and when to use modern medicine. Dr. Jennings has taught me to go a step further. Let me share with you some of the simple things I have learned.

I have already talked about the need to really think about our medications. We must ask the *why* question. We must not accept the status quo and what the culture teaches us. But I have learned from Dr. Jennings that, to state the obvious, we have brains for a reason, and I have come to believe that a lack of understanding of our "control centers" is another part of the reason that medications have become the number one killer.

Now I want to simply review some basic information about the brain physiology. If you'll hang in there with me, I'll do my best to keep it simple.

## The Brain 101

The structure of the brain that is activated by stress is called the amygdala (ah-MIG-duh-luh). Dr. Jennings equates this to the 911 center. When we're under stress, the pituitary gland acts as a 911 radio tower and puts out a call for the emergency-response team. These emergency responders are the many stress chemicals our bodies produce, including epinephrine (which raises our blood pressure and heart rate), cortisol (which regulates blood sugar), and substances called cytokines (which generate an immune response). The hippocampus, the brain's "fire chief," tells the responders when the stress is over so they can go back to the station. Controlling all these stress reactions is the limbic system.

The brain's administrator, the prefrontal cortex, controls the action. This is the thinking part of the brain, and we hope this part of your brain is well developed.

The activation of these circuits is much needed in an actual emergency situation, but what happens when this stress chemistry is "turned on" all the time? What happens when our bodies are under chronic stress? Well, the stress chemicals stay revved up. The body continues to make cytokines and epinephrine. Cytokines damage the brain cells, the neurons. This chronic inflammation affects our DNA expression. The stress centers are not being controlled correctly by the administrator. The brain's volume of neurons changes in response to stress. The thinking part of our brain, the prefrontal cortex, actually loses mass when we're under chronic stress. The stress part of the brain becomes more developed. This means we are not thinking as clearly as usual and are producing more of the stress chemicals.

The brain is bioelectric; that is, it communicates through chemicals like dopamine and serotonin, as well as through electricity. When we are thinking, electrical signals called beta waves are prevalent. In a deep sleep, delta waves are present. The brain also makes neurotropic factors—substances that stimulate growth and development. They act as brain fertilizer. Chronic stress decreases these neurotropic factors and alters the bioelectrical function of the brain. Obviously, I have grossly simplified the brain and its functions, but I wanted to give you a glimpse into the fact that the brain is definitely involved in why we take so many medications.

These chronic chemical and electrical alterations in the brain chemistry have physical consequences, including diabetes, heart attacks, increased rates of obesity, increased cholesterol and triglyceride levels, ulcers, bone loss, strokes, increased infections, inflammatory disorders, increased pain, sleep disorders, and hypertension, not to mention all the behavioral problems and "thinking issues." Needless to say, the brain can cause many of the problems that medications are intended to treat.

The stress center, the amygdala, is activated by fear. Fear from any source is not good. Television programs can incite fear, especially if one watches the evening news or violent television dramas. The amygdala is also turned on in other stressful situations, including pain, loss of sleep, dehydration, poor relationships, and basically anything that stresses an individual. I tell my patients that anything our bodies were not designed for could produce this type of stress.

Think about this for a moment. We were designed to be outside and not sit at computer terminals all day. We were designed to talk and not text. We were designed to laugh and not complain. We were designed to move and not take cars everywhere. We were designed to stay hydrated and drink water. We were designed to rest at night and not eat big meals, watch television, or stay on the computer all night. We were designed to be lean and not carry extra body weight. We were designed to serve and love one another and not fight wars. We were designed to be happy and have fun and not be depressed or anxious. We were designed to be with one another and not isolated by gaming all the time. We were designed to eat fresh fruits, vegetables, nuts, and grains, not processed and chemical-laden food. We were designed to have a relationship with our Creator that is based on love, not on fear. We were designed to be part of a family and not alone in the world. We were designed to work and be creative, not to be entertained all the time. We were designed to think for ourselves and not let others do our thinking for us. We were designed to be healthy, not to take medications.

When we are living contrary to the original design, our systems are stressed. This chronic stress affects the brain chemistry, causing alterations in gene expression as well as many other chemical reactions. This could eventually lead to disease and to a medical system that treats the symptoms derived from the altered chemical reactions with medications, which also pose a risk.

Now we're going to look at some practical solutions.

---

### USING YOUR BRAIN

Two new weight-loss medications have recently been approved by the FDA. Qsymia was the first, and the second release, Belviq, was released in July 2012. A third weight-loss medication is expected to be released soon. It is no wonder that pharmaceutical companies want to release more weight-loss drugs: in America, 30 percent of the population are now obese, and a total of 60 percent are overweight. Extra weight is a worldwide problem affecting not only adults but also children. At an estimated six dollars a pill, there is much profit to be made. This area could be a gold mine for the pharmaceutical industry, but does taking medications for obesity make sense?

Fat cells are an organ in and of themselves. This system is called the endocannabinoid system. Fat makes a host of chemicals that make us hungry, increase the stress chemicals we have alluded to, make estrogen (which increases the risk of cancer), and make inflammatory chemicals that damage the entire body, including the brain. As you can see, extra weight is not good. Many of our chronic medical problems have extra weight as the cause. The solution to date has been to make medications to block the chemistry of the fat cells. As the world continues to experience the problem of excess weight, everyone wants a quick fix.

Some medications for weight loss have been removed from the market. Ephedra-based weight-loss medications have been removed because ephedra increased the risk of abnormal heart rhythms. The first weight-loss medications, released in the 1950s and 1960s, were amphetamine-based compounds. Amphetamines speed up the metabolism.

The combination of fenfluramine and phentermine (Fen-Phen) was removed from the market because of the concern for heart valve abnormalities. Both fenfluramine and dexfenfluramine were removed in 1997. Sibutramine, another weight-loss medication, has also been removed from the market. So far there has been no quick fix.

Qsymia, one of the new medications, has as a component phentermine. The other component, topiramate, is a medication used for seizures. Some of the current known side effects of these components are increased heart rate, birth defects if used during pregnancy, and cognitive defects.

Again, when it comes to weight loss, there has been no quick fix. Extra weight changes the metabolism of the body. Now we are throwing in another chemical to "fix" the problem. That simply does not make sense to me. I expect these new medications to have a greater risk than benefit, so I am not going to recommend these medications to my patients.

You cannot suffer bad side effects from a medication you don't take. And eliminating the need for as many medications as possible should be the goal of patients and of the physicians in charge of their care.

+

# 9

# LET'S GET PRACTICAL, PART 1

*I am dying with the help of too many physicians.*
**—ALEXANDER THE GREAT**

WHEN I FIRST started writing this book, my original intent was to emphasize that we have a major problem. I believe that, thus far, we can agree on this. I believe medications are the number one cause of death. Do I have specific statistics to prove this unequivocally? No. I can only look at statistics related to many studies and reports from other sources and deduce that it is so. Will others back me up? Probably not. Yet over and over in my medical practice I have seen the dangers.

Just recently I saw a patient who earlier in the day had been given a medication to relieve pain. The prescription was to apply a salve to the back of the neck, but somehow the pharmacy instructed the nurse to place the medication in the patient's nose. Fortunately, the outcome was just an irritated nostril, but I see these types of mistakes at every level, as I have already described. In a society in which people complain of more and more symptoms, more medications will be prescribed. As we discussed in an earlier chapter, even over-the-counter medications can be dangerous. Billions and billions of prescriptions and who knows how many over-the-counter medications taken, not to mention what people are concocting on their own, create a major problem. It is not hard to realize we have the potential for mistakes at every level, adverse reactions, anaphylaxis, dependency, and death. As the numbers of medications used rise, the number of deaths will rise as well. I hope you can see the logic here.

In the media-saturated world we live in, an announcement by the head of a well-known food-service corporation can raise an immediate response. It seems that every day another YouTube video goes viral. A politician's statement goes to the world on Facebook and Twitter in seconds. I hope the information about medications and their problems will also hit the social media; then maybe serious dialogue and education will begin and will eventually result in change. If this happens, lives will be saved.

When I first began writing this book, I was going to stop writing after I exposed the problem. My office holds more material than anyone would want to read on medications and how they have been killing. Some people who read this book will likely blow off the information I have given as alarmist, but I could go on and on with examples I have seen firsthand. Now it is time to for me to get practical and offer solutions. I have a burden to perhaps help you or your loved ones avoid becoming a hidden casualty. What is so hard to fathom is that we even need so many of these medications that can so easily become lethal.

## Brenda's Story

Brenda came to see me one day in October about four years ago. Tennessee is beautiful in October. The air is crisp, and brilliant colors fill the countryside. But as Brenda and I began to talk, I could sense that she did not feel this beauty.

She was forty-three years old and the mother of two boys ages twelve and fifteen. Her main complaints were chest pain, palpitations, and shortness of breath when she was active. She carried extra weight—about 295 pounds on a five-foot-four-inch frame. My initial impression, which is so often right in the practice of medicine, was that Brenda was sad.

As we talked, I found out that she hadn't always felt this way. A few years earlier, she had felt well. But not anymore.

"Dr. Marcum," she said, "I feel overwhelmed."

I wish I could say that this was the only time I have ever heard those words.

"I do not know where to start or what to do, but I feel as if I am slowly dying," Brenda continued.

As we began our ongoing doctor-patient relationship,

Brenda's difficulties reminded me that to find a solution to a problem, we must first understand what the real problem is. In our hustle-bustle world, we frequently deal just with a symptom and move on. We want to relieve the pain, whether from a physical ailment or an emotional hurt. Brenda was being hurt on many levels. She tried to comfort her pain with food, but that was not working. The original pain, I think, started when her husband began drinking and eventually became an alcoholic. Brenda slowly lost the man who had been her best friend, and she did not know what to do. Eating helped her to feel better, and in ten years, what started as 195 pounds became 295.

As Brenda gained weight, her body chemistry changed. Fat cells, excess weight, and the endocannabinoid system (which plays a role in appetite, among other things) change the chemistry. Soon Brenda's blood pressure went up. She was prescribed a calcium channel blocker to lower her blood pressure. This medication caused some swelling in her legs, so she was given hydrochlorothiazide, a diuretic. This new medication caused her to lose potassium, so she began taking a supplement. Still her blood pressure was above normal, and an additional blood pressure medication was prescribed.

Unfortunately, Brenda became tired and quit exercising. Over the months, her blood sugar became elevated, and two medications for diabetes were added. She became more and more hungry, a side effect of blood-sugar medications, and as she ate more, her weight continued to rise.

Brenda decided to go to another doctor now that her

medication count stood at six. Her new doctor diagnosed depression and prescribed an antidepressant. This helped her mood to some extent. She continued battling these problems for a year, but the additional weight and nighttime eating were causing reflux of acid into her esophagus at night, which made it hard for her to sleep. The next prescriptions she received were for an acid-blocking medicine, as well as a sleep aid. She began sleeping a little better but was still tired.

After about six more months Brenda began to have terrible back pain and was referred to an orthopedist. A battery of tests, including an MRI, revealed musculoskeletal inflammation as the source of her pain. So, you guessed it, she was given a muscle relaxant and an anti-inflammatory medication. These helped for a short time, but as Brenda continued to gain weight, more stress was placed on her back, and she was given a narcotic medication to ease the increased pain. She also needed a bowel softener to keep her regular. Needless to say, no one stopped any of her medications.

Her change in chemistry pushed up her cholesterol and triglyceride levels, and next a statin medication was prescribed to lower the cholesterol level. Soon Brenda began to experience numbness in her lower extremities. She was sent to a neurologist, who performed another series of tests, including nerve-conduction testing. The conclusion was that her diabetes might be affecting her nerves, and yet another medicine was prescribed. Heart palpitations and chest pain prompted the addition of yet another medication just before Brenda arrived in my office that fall day. This entire painful scenario spanned three years. I now was beginning to understand why Brenda could not even notice the beautiful fall colors. She had reasons to be overwhelmed—and she was on sixteen medications.

This is hard to fathom, but I see this to similar degrees every day. Can you imagine all the interactions, the side effects, the potential for mistakes that Brenda had accumulated? Certainly all her doctors wanted to help her. But as I sat there talking to Brenda, I realized that we were not treating the cause of her physical suffering and were actually increasing her risk of death as various doctors added medication after medication to the list of prescriptions she was taking.

It took many visits and a few tears, but over time, I am glad to say, Brenda has gotten on the right path. At first she did not buy in to the treatment plan I recommended, but as her chemistry slowly changed, she realized she could alter her own chemistry by changing her thoughts, her diet, her level of activity, and her rest patterns.

Before I tell you the rest of the story, I want to emphasize once again that *there is a time and place for medications*. Sometimes the risk of the medication is worth the benefit to be gained. If I had blood clots, which could cause strokes, a blood thinner would be worth the risk. If I had a bacterial infection, an antibiotic would be worth the risk. Each individual situation must be evaluated as to the risks of a medication as well as the potential benefits.

In Brenda's situation we started by evaluating what each

medication was achieving and what problem the medication was addressing. Then we talked about the side effects, both long term and short term, of each medication. Next we discussed possible ways to change aspects of Brenda's body chemistry without taking on risk while still getting at the real causes of the problem. Brenda seemed surprised when I told her I have never seen a medication cure diabetes. She was also taken aback when we discussed her other medications and the effects they can have on the ability to think clearly and well.

Needless to say, the process was slow. It had taken years for Brenda to get as miserable as she was when she came to see me, and it would take time to make positive changes. Rome was not built in a day.

Learning where to start in helping people change is always a challenge because each of us is different. I have learned to love others, not judge them, and to point each patient to a higher power for help. Brenda began to respond as I offered her a source of hope and presented some commonsense solutions. She understood when I said, "There is a place for modern medicine, especially in the treatment of acute problems such as a heart attack. There is also a place for changing one's lifestyle, whether that means eating better, thinking better, or exercising more. But it is in the relationship with our Creator who designed us and loves us most that we get the power to change and see truth, even if the change is ever so slow. There is no pharmaceutical product that will build this relationship." This is where Brenda and I started to work.

After a month or two, Brenda began making lifestyle changes founded on how our bodies were originally designed to function. She drank more water. She started a movement program. She slowly improved her diet. As she succeeded in small ways, she felt a relationship beginning to develop with her Creator. And she increasingly began to want to change.

Soon she lost more weight, and as she got more exercise, her insulin resistance changed, and we were able to begin tapering the dosage of the diabetic medications. Her desire for calories changed, and for about six months she really dropped the weight. Her taste for processed foods changed, and as she ate fresher foods that were less processed and lower in sodium, we were able to taper the amount of blood pressure medication she needed. She quit eating big meals at night and eliminated caffeine and found she no longer needed the antacid pill or the sleep aid. Once she had lost seventy pounds, her back felt better, and she was weaned from the oxycodone, muscle relaxant, and anti-inflammatory medications. She discovered that her diet could reduce inflammation just as well as her anti-inflammatory medication could.

It was not long before she was able to stop taking a pill for her nerve pain, as the pain turned out to be a side effect of some of the other medications she was on. God was changing her thought patterns, too, as she gained confidence. I knew she would not need my help much longer when she made this statement: "Did you know that many cases of depression can be eliminated by being outside, which raises vitamin D levels and serotonin levels?" I told Brenda I thought I had heard that somewhere. It wasn't long before she was off the antidepressant, too.

To make a long story short, I no longer have to see Brenda as a patient. As of this writing, she has lost 150 pounds. She sends me articles on how people can change their chemistry by changing their diet, exercise, and thought patterns. She is in counseling with her husband and has gotten at the cause of her symptoms rather than automatically accepting treatment for her symptoms. She now realizes that healing involves more than taking medications that pose a risk.

Now, I must admit, I have presented a dramatic success story. There are many stories of people who have only begun the journey. If you are feeling overwhelmed, let me give some practical steps to possibly eliminate the risks of medications you might be taking.

First, realize that your doctor really does not want to use medication unless it is absolutely necessary. Second, realize that some medications may be worth the risks. Third, understand that genetics plays a role as well. Finally, each person is special and different, and when it comes to health plans, "one size does not fit all."

Now, let's take a closer look at those practical steps I mentioned.

## Step 1: Plug In to a Relationship with Your Creator

Developing a relationship with your Creator is an all-important step, but when you think about it, your first question might be, "How do I do this?" People connect with God in many ways. There is no set formula. I would begin by saying something like, "God, show me how to have a relationship with You and Your Son, Jesus, the way You want." God will not let you down. He has promised, "If you look for me wholeheartedly, you will find me" (Jeremiah 29:13).

If you do not know where to start, let me suggest the website heartwiseministries.org, where Jerry Arnold tells the story of how he learned to connect with God and then simply walks you through the steps. Another way is go to someone who has a relationship with God and ask, "What would you suggest?" You might get some excellent suggestions, including prayer, a quiet walk in the woods, a bike ride, an inspirational movie, an afternoon of fishing, or a worship service at a church.

Reading the Bible was an important way I started to develop my relationship with God. As I continue to read it, God teaches me how to have a relationship with Him. Other books have influenced my relationship as well. The book *More Than a Carpenter*, by Josh McDowell, really strengthened my relationship. Find out what works for you and start there. But make connecting with God a daily occurrence in whatever way works for you. Do not let the culture you live in define this relationship. Let God be God in your life. If you seek Him, He will find you, and through His Holy Spirit, He will take you where you need to go in this one-of-a-kind relationship. This relationship will also teach you truth for all aspects of your life and free you from the deceit that exists in this world. As you learn more, you will see truth about how to take care of your body and to avoid medicine when it's possible to do so. Gradually you will become more like the one you worship.

### Step 2: Learn about Your Medications

When a doctor prescribes a certain medication for you, ask him or her questions: Why are you prescribing this medication? What are the risks of this medication? Are there any drug interactions I should be aware of? Are there other ways to accomplish the same task without using a medication? What are the most common side effects you have seen?

Go to the Internet. I have found the information given on www.WebMD.com reliable. When you visit this site, go to the heading "Drugs & Supplements." On that tab there will be a section called "Find a Drug." This subsection has information on why the medication is used; its side effects, precautions, and interactions; and numerous reviews from people who have actually used the medication. A similar site is www.drugs.com. I have found this one to be reliable as well. All such sites do contain a level of bias, but these two sites are good at giving the nuts and bolts about medications. I use www.naturalnews.com as a source of information about the many natural methods available for helping to maintain good health.

If you are a type A personality who wants to know "everything there is to know" about a medication, you can consult the *Physicians' Desk Reference,* or PDR. This book is very detailed and technical. When I read this reference, I am usually scared to death to use any medication, but then I remind myself once again of the risks involved in *not* using a particular medication. Remember, many of the side effects listed in the PDR rarely occur.

The answers are out there. Make a list of all your medications and begin to learn. This is important, as medications affect every aspect of life. Learn about the most common side effects and interactions of each one. Do not depend on someone else to do this for you. Take responsibility. Most people spend more time choosing a restaurant than they do in learning about potentially toxic substances. In the next chapter I will give more information on specific medications. And perhaps someday I will write a comprehensive book about the most important details to know on every medication out there and potential ways to change your chemistry to lessen the need for the medication. For now, I want to stick with the big picture.

## Step 3: Start Making Changes Slowly

A good first change would be to begin drinking adequate water every day. Around 70 percent of your body is water, so without this vital substance, nothing works well. Every chemical reaction in the body depends on water, so not getting enough of it messes up your body chemistry. How much is enough? Take your weight and divide it by two. The result is approximately how many ounces a healthy person needs daily. If you weigh 150 pounds, you need about 75 ounces just to stay even. If you are more active, you will need more. If the weather is hot and humid, drink till your urine becomes clear. Work on this for a month until a habit is formed. The relationship that you are developing with your Creator will give you the power to continue to learn and change. Then move on to step 4.

## Step 4: Start a Movement Program

Initially your movement program may be something as simple as walking in place for a minute while swinging your arms. Then you can begin to build on this. The next week, increase that one minute to five minutes. Each week, gradually add a bit more time. Touch base with your personal doctor, of course, to make sure what you're doing is safe, but all my patients are on some type of movement program. Just as a pill changes chemistry, a movement program will change your chemistry, and more effectively than the pill, but you must move regularly. Try to build to 45 minutes of aerobics and light lifting (five pounds or so) a day. What is an aerobic activity? Walking, swimming, rowing, playing (not watching) basketball, and bicycling are all aerobic activities. Any activity that increases your heart rate is aerobic and beneficial. Sometimes I just stand in place and walk at different speeds if I have only a few minutes. You've heard the statement "Use it or lose it." If you do not use your body, you will lose it. We were designed to move. Make a chart on your calendar or use your cell phone to keep track of your movement time every day until this becomes a habit. Find someone with whom you can partner. There is power in numbers. As you move, a host of healthy chemical reactions will occur, and as long as you start slowly and gradually build up your level of physical activity, there will be no negative side effects.

## Step 5: Get Enough Rest

Rest is important. We were designed to sleep at night and also to have a longer period of rest—a Sabbath—each week. I also need vacation rest. Most people need from six to eight hours of sleep a night. Some may need a little more. A few may need less. Each body is a little different. Resting at night goes with our circadian rhythms. These are chemical rhythms in our bodies. At night these circadian chemicals diminish; they pick up again the next day. Night-shift workers have a very hard time getting rest because they are fighting the natural rhythms of the body.

Adequate and restorative rest includes allowing all parts of the body—including the brain and the digestive tract—to take a break. Try not to eat big meals at night or to stuff yourself at any time. This will help you rest better and lower your stress chemistry. Rest is a powerful healer and, again, lessens the need for certain medications. Try to rest your brain as well. We were never designed to stay up all night watching television or playing computer games or surfing the web.

One day a week, take a break from your physical and mental routines and do something entirely different on that day.

## Step 6: Start Improving Your Diet

Begin eating just a few more fresh foods and fewer processed ones. As you fill up with the fresh stuff, you will end up consuming fewer total calories.

I start my patients out by asking them to drink water and cut back on other beverages. After a month, reduce the amount of food you eat at dinner and never miss breakfast. After another month, try beginning your meals with two or three servings of fresh fruits and vegetables before you eat anything else. This fiber will help you feel full. Then eat just enough of those other foods to stay happy. The truth is, unless you stay happy with these changes, you will never stick with them. There is a place for a real feast now and then, but don't go straight to bed afterward. Take a little walk and chase the feast with some water and fiber to move the feast through the digestive tract a little quicker so rest can occur and toxic, "not so good for you" substances have less time to be absorbed.

## Step 7: Do Things That Make You Happy

Do activities you enjoy. Take a vacation. Read a book. Watch a funny movie and laugh until you cry. Go to a ball game. Visit a friend. Stay balanced. Don't forget that the relationship we talked about in step 1 is the key to staying with this program for the right reasons.

These seven practical steps are a great place to start. It may take a month or two to incorporate a step into your life. Start at the top of the list and work on the first step until it becomes a habit. These steps are not expensive. Treat each step as a prescription. To come off a medication, you will need to do something to change your chemistry naturally.

I have kept this simple for a reason. We must not become overwhelmed, or we'll never stick with it! You can read all sorts of books that go into more theory and are more complicated, but these steps are doable and are the ones I consider the most important in changing your chemistry and lessening the need for many risky medications, because, as I've said before, medications have the potential to kill.

# 10

# LET'S GET PRACTICAL, PART 2

*The art of medicine is amusing the patient while nature cures the disease.*
—VOLTAIRE

HAVE YOU EVER wished you could do something that would really make a difference? Have you seen an injustice occurring and wanted to scream? As I sat down to begin writing this chapter, I found myself wishing I were more articulate. I had just finished weekend rounds at the hospital, and that always fires me up. The first patient I saw needed a pacemaker. He was ninety-three and healthy, apart from his low heart rate of thirty-five beats per minute. This was a perfect place for modern medicine. Without the magical device called a pacemaker, this patient and many others would pass on. The next five patients were all over eighty, and all had medication issues. One fellow had taken a tranquilizer/

muscle relaxant and could barely talk to me. The next had a side effect because, although he was given the usual dose of his blood pressure medication, his kidney function had deteriorated, so the medication did not clear from his body and nearly stopped his heart. The next patient needed medications but had decided to spend his money on alcohol instead. These days I spend more time reviewing medications and trying to figure out what the patients are actually doing with their medications than anything else. I feel as if I have become a medication detective. And I have certainly learned that the less medicine I prescribe, the less the likelihood there is for error at every level.

In this chapter, I want to give some more practical ways you might be able to come off some medications. I cannot go over every single medication, but I would like to work from the most-prescribed-medication list I give in Appendix D. The top ten are as follows: hydrocodone, for pain; simvastatin (brand name Zocor), for high cholesterol; lisinopril, for high blood pressure; amlodipine (brand name Norvasc), for high blood pressure; omeprazole (brand name Prilosec), to block stomach acid; azithromycin and amoxicillin, for bacterial infections; metformin (brand name Glucophage), to lower blood sugar; and hydrochlorothiazide, another medication for blood pressure. I am leaving out one top-ten medication, Synthroid, which is used to treat low levels of thyroid hormone. I am going to add in sleep medications, weight-loss medications, diuretics, chemotherapy medications, medications for inflammation, and depression medications.

This list will cover many of the medications people are on and give some practical and commonsense suggestions for how it might be possible to lower the dose of a medication or even come off a medication or two. Keeping it simple is important—as is checking with your physician before stopping any medication.

## Pain Medications

More and more people are dying from overdoses, dangerous drug interactions, and accidents resulting from impaired thinking caused by pain medications. The numbers are not completely reported. How many traffic accidents, drownings, or even homicides can be linked in some way to narcotics?

As the number of pharmaceutical producers and sales of these medications continues to rise dramatically, the death rate from problems associated with this type of medication will continue to increase. Earlier, when I quoted articles that described the issue in terms of the number of people that medicines kill, narcotics-related deaths were not even factored into the equation.

How do you come off these potentially dangerous and addictive medications? The seven steps in chapter 9 are a great place to start. You should also identify why you are using painkillers. Some people have legitimate medical reasons for taking medications for pain. But in other cases, people are taking pain medications for conditions that could be treated in other, safer ways to alleviate the cause of their pain.

One example would be a bad back that could be surgically repaired or treated with physical therapy or manipulation. One of my patients has been taking medications for back pain for twenty years. She has an implanted narcotic pump and also takes narcotic pills. When I asked her if she had ever had the cause of her pain evaluated, she told me about the four-plus back operations she had undergone. She came to me because she had been having heart attacks and heart problems for years. But the pain that came from her heart problems had been undetected, and this resulted in permanent damage to her heart. I am positive the heavy doses of narcotics masked the symptoms of her heart disease. I wonder whether something more could have been done twenty years ago to not only help her heart but also to keep her from using so many pain medications.

Some pain is caused and aggravated by inflammation. As I've mentioned before, drinking more water, getting enough rest, eating a more plant-based diet, and eating certain foods can help with inflammation. We know that a regular exercise program helps with pain by increasing the natural painkiller endorphin. Sometimes laughter really is the best medicine, because it triggers the release of endorphins that can help alleviate pain.[1]

Of course, much pain is caused by life in general. You may be trying to escape difficult or painful circumstances, and narcotics numb the senses so you can forget the pains of life for a while. If you are in this type of pain, I encourage you to obtain professional help and turn to the ultimate Physician for answers.

## Cholesterol-Lowering Medications

Everyone has heard about cholesterol and its association with cardiovascular disease. Statins, a class of cholesterol-lowering medications, are among the most prescribed medications in the world. Unfortunately, these medications can also damage the liver and muscles. There have also been deaths associated with the statin class of cholesterol-lowering drugs.

To potentially get off this medication, ask your doctor to evaluate your overall risk first. When the risk for my patients is low, I try to get them to move toward a plant-based diet and make exercise a prescription. Animals and animal products contain cholesterol. One of the most effective ways to lower your levels is simply not to eat foods with cholesterol in them. Certain high-fiber foods can actually help to lower cholesterol levels. Do not forget that exercise changes your chemistry greatly, but to benefit from it, you need to do it on a regular basis.

With much of the world eating less healthfully and living under more stress than ever, cholesterol levels will continue to rise. The number of prescriptions for statins will continue to rise. And the rate of complications, including deaths, will rise as well.

## Blood Pressure Medications

Many people are taking blood pressure medications. High blood pressure, or hypertension, has been called the "silent killer" because it can damage the blood vessels and increase the risk of heart attack, stroke, and renal (kidney) disease. I often see people become unsteady and fall when their blood pressure drops too much from blood pressure medications. If you become dehydrated while on these medications, your blood pressure can drop. This drop could cause a fainting spell, and if you are doing something like driving a car or taking a shower, a "bonk" on the head or a broken hip—or worse—would be a big deal.

Three factors have really caused an epidemic of blood pressure problems: too much salt in the diet (often from eating too much processed food), carrying too much weight (up to 60 percent of Americans are overweight), and inactivity (we were designed to move, not just sit on the couch). Along with this rise in blood pressure problems have come more prescriptions—and, consequently, more problems. I have not seen many cases in which blood pressure medications have directly caused a death, but I have seen instances in which people have fallen or passed out when their blood pressure has become too low as a result of those medications.

How do you get off a blood pressure medication? Get at the cause. If you are too heavy, work on getting to a healthy weight. If you eat too much salted food, pick up more fresh fruits and veggies. If you tend to sit around, start moving. If you have sleep apnea, which causes high blood pressure, wear a sleep mask and lose weight. If you are stressed because your next-door neighbor is throwing trash into your yard, find a way to resolve the conflict.

If the cause can be remedied, your doctor would be more

than happy to give you a trial period off the medication and monitor your blood pressure. Of course, some people need to take a blood pressure medication even when they have dealt with their various stressors. We cannot change our genetics yet, but the possibility of taking a lower dose of the medication or even taking one less medication will lower the medicine-related risks.

## Acid-Blocking Medications

Medications that block acid in the stomach are commonly used for ulcers and reflux problems. Nexium, Prilosec, Pepcid, and Tagamet are a few of the names under which these acid-blocking medications are sold. Unfortunately, these medications can block the absorption of other medications that depend on a normal pH (acid/alkaline) balance. Some have been associated with osteoporosis-related fractures. These medications were designed to be used for only short periods of time because they can mask the symptoms of more serious problems, such as stomach cancer.

Mary had been on acid-blocking medications for twenty years. She broke her hip the day after Thanksgiving 2007. Complications developed, including a blood clot in one of her calves, which moved to her lungs. This cascade of events led to her death. One must wonder whether the prolonged use of acid-blocking medications might have contributed to the development of osteoporosis and the hip fracture, as well as this series of events.

In limiting these medications, I would suggest asking a few questions: *Why am I on this medication? Is it for over-production of acid in my case? How can I lower acid production naturally?*

Caffeine, which 90 percent of Americans ingest daily, has been associated with acid production. Other stressors include the use of cigarettes and failure to drink enough water. These could trigger extra acid formation. Another biggie is the protein-laden, fat-filled meal we tend to eat at night. The stomach has to produce additional acid to digest this late meal. Then the victim goes to bed, making it easy for the acid to move into the esophagus, causing reflux. This is no fun at all.

It might be possible for a person to eliminate the need for this type of medication just by eating lighter meals at night, avoiding hard-to-digest foods, cutting back on caffeine, and drinking more water.

Finally, I would recommend lowering stress in one's life, whatever this might entail for the patient. When the body is under stress, it produces more acid to digest nutrients needed to deal with the perceived stress.

## Antibiotics

Antibiotics are used to fight bacterial infections. They are prescribed to the young and old alike. They have helped save many lives over the years, and I personally have seen them do much good during my twenty-plus years in medicine. So, why would I write about coming off these medications? I'm not. But I am suggesting that whenever possible, you avoiding taking them. Earlier I cited statistics about how many antibiotic prescriptions are written that just are not needed.

What are the risks of taking an antibiotic? First, an anaphylactic reaction to an antibiotic can kill you. Second, as a society takes more and more antibiotics, organisms that are resistant to specific medications can develop. Then the antibiotics are no longer able to destroy them. Overuse of antibiotics facilitates the development of these resistant organisms.

Third, antibiotics can be toxic to organs such as the kidneys. Again, I am not suggesting that you quit taking antibiotics. I am merely suggesting that you take them only when they are really needed. Many infections are caused by viruses. And though these infections are unpleasant while they last, in many instances, your own immune system will take care of them, and they will run the course on their own. Taking an antibiotic does no good for this type of infection.

Ask your doctor if an antibiotic is really needed for your upper respiratory infection. Often children with earaches can be spared the use of antibiotics as well. The statistics I shared earlier suggest many antibiotics are prescribed not because they are needed but because physicians feel their patients want the medication. If we can lessen the use of antibiotics, we can also lessen the risks associated with using them.

## Diabetes Medications

There are several types of diabetes. Type 1 diabetics need insulin, and this type of diabetes, again, is clearly a place for modern medicine. But the vast majority of people with diabetes have type 2 diabetes, sometimes called insulin-resistant diabetes. This type of diabetes has a complex physiology, but the basic problem is too much fat—in the diet and in the body. Type 2 diabetes damages the blood vessels and organs throughout the body.

I have never seen a medication cure type 2 diabetes. Often medications used to treat this type of diabetes act as growth hormones in the body and may increase the appetite of the person taking them. Increased appetite often means increased food consumption, which leads to increased weight—and, well, you get the picture. Some diabetes medications used over the years have been shown to be toxic. I have seen people die from medications used to lower blood sugar, especially when the blood sugar level goes too low. This can occur when the body does not break down the medication or when an overdose occurs. Elderly people in a nursing home sometimes get sick and do not eat or drink enough and yet are still given their medications for type 2 diabetes. This leads to complications.

How might a person get off these medications? First, he or she should cut back on the amount of fat in the body by eating a healthy diet. Then he or she should add exercise, exercise, and more exercise. If people are willing to work hard at this, they often can be tapered off their medications for type 2 diabetes.

## Sleep Medications

More and more patients are on medications to help them sleep. Medications sold under names such as Ambien, Halcion, Lunesta, and Restoril are a few on the market. One of my patients, an eighty-year-old former minister, related that he was recently in the hospital and having a hard time getting to sleep. He received a sleep aid, and the next thing he remembered was waking up in the hospital parking lot naked. I doubt he will take a sleep aid again anytime soon.

Sleep medications do not help a person live longer, and a few studies have shown that persons who take them regularly have cognitive dysfunction; in other words, they aren't quite as mentally sharp as before they began using the medication. These medications were originally approved for only short-term use, never for prolonged use. They are addictive. There are always interactions with other medications and alcohol. These medicines essentially just knock you out.

When people tell me they want to stop taking a sleep medicine, my initial approach is to find out why they do not sleep well to begin with. Is it related to a medical condition such as sleep apnea or an enlarged prostate that may be causing them to wake up frequently during the night? Other medical conditions, including cardiovascular disease, asthma, cancer, and chronic pain, can also cause insomnia.

Are they taking in stimulants such as caffeine or energy drinks? Are they using drugs or alcohol? One of the easiest patients I helped was a young woman who could not sleep. The problem was the stimulant in her weight-loss medications. Some people can't sleep because their bodies are busy digesting a big meal at night. Others are just too stimulated from watching television—too much violence, too much news. Their minds are overloaded and cannot rest. Insomnia must be thought of as a symptom. The key to their getting off a sleep medication is to find out why they were not sleeping well in the first place. First, make sure you do not have a medical condition that is contributing to your difficulty sleeping.

A natural supplement called melatonin sometimes helps. Melatonin is a hormone released by the pineal gland in the brain. One of its functions is to regulate the sleep-wake cycle. As people age, the amount of this hormone the brain releases may decrease. Melatonin is available as a supplement, and some people may find it helpful. A regular exercise program is also useful in helping people come off sleep aids.

Is it possible to die from a sleep aid? Yes. One study has reported that people who were prescribed one to 18 doses a year had a 3.5 times greater risk of death than those who do not use sleep aids.[2]

Michael Jackson suffered from insomnia and desperately wanted to sleep. He went to medicinal extremes, using the anesthetic agent propofol for sleep. His death shocked the world.

## Weight-Loss Medications

If I were banging my head on the wall, the real solution would not be to take morphine to take the pain away. The real solution would be to quit banging my head on the wall. That seems obvious, doesn't it? So, why take a medication that involves risk? We have spoken about the weight-loss medication Fen-Phen and the damage it did to heart valves before it was removed from the market. Most weight-loss medications have stimulants that cause side effects. These medications are not made for the long haul. Most put the cardiovascular system at risk and, in addition, are not inexpensive.

How do you come off these medications? Stop taking them. *Stop taking them now.* Learn how to eat healthy. Move your body regularly. And pray for help to live a healthier lifestyle.

## Diuretics

Diuretics are used to remove fluid from the body and are frequently used when patients have heart failure or kidney failure. However, I also see them used extensively for swelling in the legs. This is frequently brought on by too much salt in the diet. Salt is hidden in preserved and packaged foods, and the average person eats way too much of these and is often too quick to reach for the salt shaker at meals—even before tasting what's on his or her plate.

Medicines sold under such names as hydrochlorothiazide, Lasix, Demadex, chlorthalidone, and Bumex are a few of these commonly used. These medications are not smart enough to pull fluid only from the legs and can cause the body to lose important electrolytes and become dehydrated, which hurts the function of the kidneys.

I have seen persons develop renal failure and die because they continued to take their diuretics but were not eating or drinking. I have also seen lethal heart rhythms occur when the potassium level became too low from the pills' effects.

Ask your doctor why you are taking a diuretic. If it's just for fluid in the legs, try cutting your salt intake. Wearing compression stockings or elevating your legs when you are sitting might help move fluid to the larger veins so it can be carried away. A movement program will also improve the function of the veins. This could start with simply walking in place and moving your arms up and down for one minute. Many of my patients have come off diuretics by making these simple changes, which get at the cause of the problem rather than just treating another symptom.

## Chemotherapy Drugs

The medications used in chemotherapy are powerful and damage good cells as well as cancer cells. The bone-marrow cells—which make cells to fight infections, help our blood to clot, and also carry oxygen—may be damaged. As anyone who has been on chemotherapy can attest, these medications are toxic. "If the cancer doesn't kill you, the chemo will" is a phrase I have heard more than once.

Do your best to avoid these medications by lowering your risk of cancer in the first place. Avoid prolonged exposure to carcinogens such as cigarettes. Keep your body weight in a healthy range. (This will lower your exposure to estrogen, which contributes to the development of some cancers.) Do not burn your skin through prolonged exposure to sunlight. Increase your consumption of fiber (fruits and veggies) and lower your consumption of meat and processed foods. (This will limit the intestinal tract's exposure to carcinogens and lower the risk of colon cancer.)

Early detection is also important. Get the screening exams. Have a colonoscopy, prostate check or mammogram, and skin exam. If you are not feeling well, don't just wait for the feeling to go away; get checked out.

Chemotherapy is one of the most dangerous classes of medication. Do all you can to avoid the need for it.

## Nonsteroidal Anti-Inflammatory Medications

Nonsteroidal anti-inflammatory drugs (NSAIDs) would include those such as Advil, Ecotrin, Naprosyn, Mobic, Voltaren, and Daypro. Vioxx used to be on the list but, as we discussed earlier, was removed because of its link to increased risk for heart attack. This class of medications treats inflammation and is being used for all types of aches and pains. These medications do work; however, there could be side effects. The number one cause of fatal gastrointestinal bleeding is this class of medications.

How might you come off NSAIDs? First, assess the level of pain for which the drug is being used. Many people are self-medicating because they can buy this medication over the counter. But in many cases, they are using way too much to control their pain. I know of one patient who kept popping NSAIDs until he bled to death from a peptic ulcer. He would have been better off with a little pain or adding another medicine that had a different list of side effects.

Next, try other remedies that may help inflammation, such as adequate hydration (drinking enough water) and avoiding heavily processed foods, which can be very fattening and therefore can trigger inflammation. Eat more veggies and foods high in omega-3 fatty acids, such as fish, whole grains, olive oil, and garlic. Exercise and daily stretching might be valuable and enable you to eliminate this type of medication. Getting adequate rest will also help to reduce inflammation.

Also, do not forget to get at the cause of the inflammation if possible. If lifting heavy weights causes inflammation, stop lifting heavy weights and find another way to get fit. If a certain pair of shoes rubs on your feet, wear different shoes. If you have a toothache, see a dentist. If you have headaches from staying up too late unnecessarily, get more rest. I think you get the picture about eliminating, whenever possible, any causes of the inflammation for which you are using the medicine.

Of course, some people, especially those with arthritis, might need this class of medications. The pain and subsequent chemical reactions from this stressor might be a greater risk than the medication itself. But it's important to monitor the side effects, and I would recommend also doing everything else possible to lower the inflammatory burden on the body. This can help to lower the dependence on medicines and maybe lower the risk of a lethal side effect.

## Medications for Depression

It has been estimated that one in four individuals has a mental health problem. At the top of the list of these problems is clinical depression. There is no blood test to diagnose depression. It is a clinical diagnosis made after a physician has evaluated the patient in light of a set of specific symptoms. Common medicines used for depression include those sold under such names as Lexapro, Celexa, Prozac, Effexor, Cymbalta, Paxil, and Zoloft, to name just a few. All antidepressant medications have the potential to be lethal. They are especially dangerous when used in conjunction with alcohol.

How might you be able to come off this type of medication? First make sure the diagnosis of clinical depression is correct. There are medical conditions such as hypothyroidism, chronic pain, deficiencies in the diet, and sleep apnea, to name a few, that must be eliminated as causes and treated if necessary. Situational depression may look like clinical depression but is related to a life event such as a death or loss of a job. Helping a person heal from such an event simply by being a good friend may make the use of long-term medication unnecessary.

There are other ways to change the brain chemistry in the same way an antidepressant medication does but without the same risks. Getting out in the sunlight or taking a supplement can boost your vitamin D level, which is critical for the production of the brain chemical serotonin. Exercise can boost your mood by increasing the production of endorphins. A diet with antioxidants and omega-3 fatty acids can improve brain function.

Finally, I believe serving others, worshiping God, taking time to smell the roses, enjoying pets, laughing, and getting sufficient rest can improve brain function as well.

With the steady rise in depression, I look at the world we live in and wonder, *What has gone wrong?* What is it about how we are living that alters our brain chemistry and produces the symptoms of depression? If we can answer this question, there is a chance to come off the medication.

Don't forget: some people need medications, as their genetics cause the problem; however, many can come off these medications under a doctor's supervision.

# 11

# THE REST OF THE STORY

*Learn from the past. Live for the present. Long for the future.*
—JAMES L. MARCUM, MD

I LIKE THE ACCOUNT of the preacher who was visiting the home of a distraught parishioner. The man was clearly in emotional pain; he was fearful and agitated and had been so for several weeks. The preacher asked, "What's the problem, my friend? You seem so upset."

"Upset?" the man cried. "Of course I'm upset! Haven't you seen the state of the world today? Haven't you seen the suffering, the pain, the anguish that so many are experiencing? Any caring person would be upset!"

The minister nodded slowly, then handed the man his Bible. "Here," he said, "this will help."

"The Bible?" the churchgoer scoffed. "I know all about

the Ten Commandments, the Beatitudes, and the story of Jonah. How are they supposed to ease my worry?"

The preacher flipped through the pages. "You need to read right *here*."

"Revelation?" the man gasped. "The last book in the Bible? Why?"

The minister looked deeply into the eyes of his parishioner. "You may have noticed that I'm not as distraught as you are about life, about sin, and about the future. The reason is, I've read these passages. They explain what's coming. They tell us the rest of the story, and when you read these words, the future looks bright indeed. That gives me hope."

Please believe me when I say that I would never, *ever* say the things I said in the first half of this book if I didn't understand what I'm about to tell you in the next few pages. I would never suggest that the prescription medicines you are taking are dangerous and potentially damaging to your long-term health if I didn't know, conclusively, what the rest of the story can be for you and me. I know beyond a doubt that there are powerful alternatives we can put to work as we try to gain and maintain optimum health. Ending my book here would be like snatching the crutches from a woman with a broken leg before explaining that injured legs will heal and she will be able to walk again.

So, please stay with me. I know how much better it can get for you and for me *if* we make some changes in our lives. I've discovered that our future is brightest when we seriously consider, and then put into action, the principles of optimum health that are deeply embedded in the past we all share. We must learn from the past and live in the present but look forward to a better future.

## A New Perspective

Many people are surprised to learn that I consider the Bible to be the greatest health manual ever written. I can't say that I blame them. After all, no one recalls reading anything about cures for the common cold, effective ways to battle obesity, or the way changing your diet can protect you against cancer. Nowhere tucked in the pages of Scripture has anyone found a prescription for heart disease or an ancient medical study throwing new light on the causes and cures of diabetes.

However, I have discovered that the Bible addresses every one of these modern diseases in some very specific ways. You just have to shift your perspective a little. That's what happened to me when I became a doctor. I started seeing the world from a decidedly medical angle. I began to ask myself, *Why didn't God warn us about what was coming? Why didn't He prepare us for these terrible diseases that plague us? Why didn't He tell us what we needed to do to avoid them?*

Slowly, over time, I began to realize that He did! Interestingly, that conclusion didn't come from God's Word but from the scientific community. As I learned the healing craft, I started seeing patterns that sounded vaguely familiar. It was as if I'd heard this information before, as if I'd read about the connection between a particular activity and enjoying health benefits.

Then one day the lights came on. I *had* heard these things before—in church, in the Bible, in the book of Genesis. I realized that God hadn't left us to fend for ourselves when it comes to building and maintaining optimum health. There *were* heaven-ordained ways to bypass most illnesses. There *were* ways to reduce our dependence on the medical profession, hospitals, and CAT scans. We could, indeed, bring healing to our bodies without the invasive and often deadly intervention of the latest and greatest medical procedures. We could be healthy in spite of heredity, environment, and past errors in judgment. We could, indeed, live drug free.

This new perspective for health requires two fundamental beliefs: first, that the Creator God not only brought man and woman into existence but also created a specific environment that would ensure they lived, literally, forever. Second, that the further away we move from that environment and the principles that govern it, the more stress we have to deal with and the sicker we become.

Of course, many people have asked me, "How do you know the Bible is true?" As you might imagine, it is beyond the scope of this book to get into this discussion in any detail. But as I looked at the evidence—the biblical prophecies, the geology of the earth, the eye-witness accounts, and science— I came to the conclusion that the Bible is true and is the Word of God. I encourage everyone to examine the evidence. I found the book *More Than a Carpenter* by Josh McDowell very helpful. And although the ways the Bible is interpreted may vary, the longer I live and see God working, the more my faith in the Bible is strengthened.

If you do not believe in the Bible, I encourage you to look at its principles and see whether there is science behind those principles. Hear me out, and then examine the evidence for yourself, as I have. There is no harm in doing this. Even if you end up disagreeing with my conclusions, I think you will find the discussion that follows helpful in perhaps avoiding the dangers of the medications we have looked at in previous chapters.

I found that within the verdant boundaries of the Garden of Eden, God made available to Adam and Eve—and all future human beings—everything that was needed to enjoy life eternal. Most of us forget that. But by understanding the important connection between who we are (God's created children) and how we are to live (a lifestyle designed by that same God), we can open the door to some incredible insights.

God didn't change the rules regulating how to enjoy optimum health when selfishness entered the scene. Those rules didn't stop operating simply because we decided that appetite was more important than common sense or that sickness is the result of not taking enough of the right pills or that modern medicine knows more about us than God does. The terrible truth is that we—first Adam and Eve, and then every future generation—put ourselves in charge of ourselves. We're paying a terrible price for that arrogance.

However, God is all about second chances. That's what

He's offering to us today. We can't go back to the way it used to be, but we can move in a direction toward what life was like then. Yes, the scenery has changed dramatically, but the God-given principles related to health have not.

So, what was this environment designed specifically to assure human beings optimum health and longevity? Let's find out.

## Laws of Health

"Here we go again!" I can hear you saying. "A religion-based scientist talking about *laws*. I'd much rather hear you talk about grace and forgiveness and how Jesus died for me. Besides, didn't Christ spend most of His ministry on earth railing against the religious 'laws' of His time?"

Absolutely, especially those that ran contrary to the rules and regulations He'd put in place long before Bethlehem. By the time He physically arrived on the scene, those religious laws had been so distorted that no one could figure them out—especially the hapless population required to follow them.

Laws, even biblical ones, have a bad habit of being warped and bent in order to comfortably fit a perceived human need or requirement. Let's face it: many of us obey laws only to the point where they don't get in our way. Ask any driver who's late to work.

That same thing has happened to the laws of health that the Creator God formed right along with human beings during Creation. Only this time it's not the threat of getting to work late or losing a paycheck that motivates our departure from the principles we know to be right. Today it's appetite, habit, tradition, modern medicine, modern science, and that all-important, all-knowing, all-powerful media on which we so desperately depend. We seem to have no problem at all bending God's Creation laws to fit within those dangerous parameters.

However, the fact that we don't believe a law exists—or can't explain it—doesn't mean the law is not in operation. Jump off a cliff, and the law of gravity guarantees that you're going to enjoy a short and thrilling drop to the rocks below. You might not know how to explain what gravity is. You might not even believe that it exists or that you're actually a victim of it. But the law exists, and your deadly fall is proof.

The laws of health God set up in Eden are in full operation today, just as they were for Adam and Eve. However, for whatever reasons, very few of us bother to abide by them. But that doesn't change the fact that they are up and running and that we will reap the unpleasant results of breaking them.

So, if you'll forgive me, I'd like to remind you of those laws. I think you'll discover, as I have, that ignoring them doesn't change their potency. Understanding them might help you avoid a medication or a dangerous side effect. It is safer, whenever possible, to change the body's chemistry by following these laws.

Let's take a stroll through Creation week and see what God had in mind when He spoke this world—and us—into existence.

## Day 1: Light (Setting the Stage for Health)

"Formless and empty." That's how my New International Version of the Bible describes this world on the first day of Creation. It also says that the surface was covered by "darkness" (see Genesis 1:2).

Have you ever felt that way? I have! Ignoring God's principles makes you *feel* just like the uncreated world *looked*—awash with dark thoughts and devoid of purpose. You've tried everything to make yourself feel better, think better, and even act better. But nothing seems to work.

That's why God's very first command offers such hope. He looked at this dark, swirling mess that was our earth and spoke four simple words: "Let there be light" (Genesis 1:3).

I've got to tell you, things—amazing things—happen when God speaks. Suddenly, for the first time, this "dark emptiness" we now call home began to change. Hollywood's most skillful special-effects artists could never do it justice. God did more than make light. He made everything that followed possible.

Could there be a more healing message that I could give a sick person today? I don't care how old you are. I don't care what you've done to yourself in the years leading up to now. I don't care if you're at death's door. You can be better! You can experience improvement. You can be stronger, more alive, than you are at this moment. The answer isn't found in modern medicine. Long-term healing requires that the Spirit of God "hover" over your life to bring light to your mind and teach you what you need to know about health. *Better health is possible!*

Do you want proof?

Surgeon Caldwell Esselstyn, MD, of the famed Cleveland Clinic, studied two dozen heart disease patients who'd been told by their physicians to "go home and prepare for death" and tried something radical. He changed their diets. He and his wife changed their diets too. To what? To the types of plant-based foods that Adam and Eve ate in the Garden of Eden. All who stayed on the program recovered, and most are still alive today, almost twenty-five years later.

Did these precious people suddenly become religious and begin attending church? Was their new diet labeled "biblical"? No. They simply, unknowingly, started living by the laws of health God set in motion a very long time ago. They put their trust in ancient laws they didn't fully understand. But something amazing happened. They moved from the darkness of mostly self-inflicted damage to their cardiovascular systems into the light of the healing power generated by God's laws of health.

In his bestselling book, *Prevent and Reverse Heart Disease*, Dr. Esselstyn concludes, "I believe that coronary artery disease is preventable, and that even after it is under way, its progress can be stopped, its insidious effects reversed. I believe, and my work over the past twenty years has demonstrated, that all this can be accomplished without expensive mechanical intervention and with minimal use of drugs. The key lies in nutrition."[1]

That's "light" if I've ever seen it!

*Tiger on the Path*

Before I go any further, let me spend a moment talking to you about stress. We all know what it is. You're walking along a jungle path and suddenly, there in front of you, is a tiger ready to pounce. What happens next is classic stress—here's the short list:

1. Your heart rate soars, delivering a burst of added oxygen to brain and muscles so you can think and act quickly.
2. Your digestion stops, so that all your energies can be utilized by your fight-or-flight mechanisms.
3. Your breathing becomes shallow but rapid, assuring a rich supply of oxygen to the blood.
4. Your pupils dilate so you can see even in low-light situations.
5. Your blood thickens in preparation for possible injury so you won't bleed out.

In other words, your whole body goes on high alert. You're ready to do whatever it takes to escape the situation and live to see another day. When the big cat decides that you probably aren't as tasty as you look and moves on, you're left drenched with sweat and trembling uncontrollably.

Slowly, all the symptoms reverse themselves. You shake your head, thank whatever deity you believe in that you're still in one piece, and move on down the path, promising yourself that tomorrow you'll find another way to the village.

Stress is our bodies' way of preparing for the unexpected, and usually this is a good thing. However, it is an altered state. In that condition, our bodies are not functioning normally and are certainly not concerned about long-term health. They just want to keep us alive for the next few minutes.

These days, most of us don't face tigers on our paths. We face belligerent bosses, defiant children, unresponsive spouses, or uncaring neighbors. We deal with traffic jams, road rage, terrorism, wars, financial meltdowns, foreclosures, and violent scenes on TV or the silver screen. Yet our bodies respond in very much the same ways.

That's the problem. When our bodies are experiencing mental or physical stress, they cannot utilize all the good things we do for our health. Our healthy diets, great exercise programs, and brain-strengthening mental stimulations take a backseat to the simple act of survival. That's why chronically stressed people experience much less improvement in their well-being after adopting sound health principles—even biblical ones. These unfortunate individuals usually then turn around and start attacking those principles, insisting that they're useless. Their bodies are just so busy facing down the "tigers" in their lives—they're so busy living in that altered state—that the power of making healthy choices can't fully operate. Stress is the wild card of health; it's the loose cannon on the deck of the storm-tossed ship trying to do battle with the wind, the waves, and the enemy all at the same time.

So, it's vital that any journey to optimum health begin with a journey inward to how we react to our world and the things happening to us. There are many wonderful books written on this subject. I recommend *Could It Be This Simple?: A Biblical Model for Healing the Mind*, by my friend Dr. Timothy R. Jennings.

That said, let's continue examining what God had in mind when He turned the void into beauty during Creation week, as recorded in Genesis 1. Let's look at another principle that may protect us from the need for dangerous medications.

## Day 2: Air and Water

The second day of Creation saw the introduction of vital elements of optimum health: air and water. More to the point, *fresh* air and *clean* water.

### Air

"Wait a minute, Dr. Marcum," I can hear you say. "Are you telling me that I could be sick because I'm not breathing right?"

Air is around 20 percent oxygen. Every one of your more than 100 trillion cells must receive a steady, fresh supply of oxygen, or it will die. Breathing is how that oxygen gets into your lungs, where it is then transferred to the red blood cells. So, you tell me. Can a person be healthy if he or she doesn't breathe right?

That's why I recommend to my patients that they spend a few minutes every day drawing in a few slow, deep breaths of air (as unpolluted as possible).

Another way to assure an adequate supply of oxygen in the body is through regular exercise. Walking, jogging, climbing stairs—anything that gets your heart pumping just a little faster than normal and gets your breath rate elevated a bit—is flooding your body with oxygen. This type of activity opens up blood vessels and speeds those oxygen-rich red blood cells on their rounds. I'm sorry, but sitting in front of a computer, watching television, or playing video games doesn't qualify as exercise, no matter how interesting or exciting the content may be.

Here's a little "air inventory" you can take right now to see if you are encouraging or discouraging healthful air intake:

- If you are sitting, is your spine straight? Are your shoulders squared? Good posture encourages deeper breathing and better oxygen intake.
- Is your breathing shallow or deep? Deeper breaths are better.
- Do either your clothes or your chair restrict your breathing in any way?
- Is your room well ventilated with fresh air, or is it closed and stuffy? Do you have oxygen-producing houseplants sprinkled about your humble abode or office space? Have you (or will you) exercise today?
- Are you eating healthy foods? A high-fat meal or snack reduces your blood's ability to carry oxygen.
- Have you taken a break during the past two hours to get up and move about for a few minutes?

- Are you stressed out all the time and finding yourself breathing too fast?
- Are you exposed to cigarette smoke or other toxic fumes?

God made air for a reason: it is critical to optimum health. When our bodies don't get sufficient oxygen, stress and its damaging chemical reactions ensue. Don't neglect oxygen. This seems so basic and yet is so important.

## Water

You remember water, don't you? It's what we all drank before we decided to teach the world to sing. Forcing our bodies to operate with insufficient fluids is like trying to wash the dinner dishes in a cupful of water. When you don't introduce enough water, your systems must excrete wastes in much more concentrated forms, creating body odor, bad breath, and stinky urine. Those are just the obvious results.

But there are some much more serious side effects of limiting your water intake. I can truthfully say that if my patients drank as much water each day as they drink coffee, tea, milk, alcoholic beverages, and colas, a lot fewer of them would have to remain my patients.

Every chemical reaction that takes place in the human body—and there are countless numbers of them each day— takes place in a water-based environment. Every one! When we become dehydrated—a condition that plagues a majority of people in most countries—these reactions are hindered. The transfer of toxins out of our bodies grinds to a slower and slower pace, leaving waste material languishing deep in our bodily systems. I don't mean to gross you out, but imagine what would happen if you decided to flush your toilet only a couple of times a week. You get the idea.

The good news is that a whole-food, plant-based diet (more on this later) can greatly increase the amount of water in your body since these foods are primarily made up of water. You're putting in a fresh supply every time you eat that type of food. But you still need to keep fresh, clean drinking water handy to remain well hydrated.

Water is also a natural blood thinner. It's a no-fat, no-sugar, no-calories wonder, and the Creator made sure there was an abundant supply of it before animals or humans showed up. We need to carry on that tradition. If you are adequately hydrated, the dangers of medications can be minimized. Medications do not work as intended in a "dry" state. When you are adequately hydrated, you will also think better. Remember the characters in books you've read or movies you've seen who are stranded somewhere without enough water? Sooner or later, they start seeing things that aren't there. The last time I was dehydrated, I could not even form a thought.

If you do not drink enough water, a chemical change will take place in your body. This may lead to a symptom of one kind or another, which may lead to a medication, which may lead to a risk of other problems, when the real problem was simply not drinking enough water to enable your body to function properly.

## Day 3: Powerful, Health-Building Plants

Take a nice patch of soil; add seeds, water, and sunshine; and soon you'll have yourself the most powerful medicines available on this planet.

Day three of Creation week saw the stocking of God's medicine cabinet. In it He placed grains, roots, blossoms, veggies, fruits, nuts, beans, and all the other amazing items calling out to those who breeze by the grocery store's produce section on their way to the meat counter.

Today, modern science seems to be falling all over itself in a rush to convince us of the power of plants. The incredible 2011 film documentary *Forks over Knives* brought this message home to the masses. No longer do we need to take God's word for it (which is kind of sad, when you think about it). Now we can look to science for conclusive proof that God knew what He was doing when He played farmer on day three.

One of the damaging elements to the human cardiovascular systems is the eating of animal products. Why? Fat.

One of the most healing elements to the human cardiovascular system is the eating of whole plant foods. Why? Fiber.

Fat, along with cholesterol, calcium, and few other ingredients, is what generates the formation of plaque within your arteries. Plaque is that sticky, gooey stuff that builds up on arterial walls, then becomes brittle and stiff. This not only reduces blood flow in those areas, thus increasing blood pressure (think of the force necessary to move water through a pinched water hose), it also produces a perfect place for a clot to form. When no blood gets through, whatever is downstream dies. That could be your heart (heart attack) or your brain (stroke). Fat also encourages a process called oxidation, a chemical change that damages the blood vessels.

Fiber, on the other hand, helps the body. It can actually improve bowel function, does not contain fat, and makes you feel full. Many high-fiber foods are good antioxidants, which help reverse the dangerous chemical reaction of oxidation I mentioned in the last paragraph.

Think of fiber as millions of tiny delivery vans entering your system with their loads of nutrients fresh from the plants you just ate. After off-loading their cargo in the right place at the right time, these vans, now empty, begin a second life as garbage trucks, collecting waste materials such as plaque, various toxins, dead cells, and excess hormones—to name just a few—and carrying them through your alimentary canal, where they are eventually eliminated. Animal products contain loads of fat and zero fiber. All problem. No solution.

Allow me to get a little technical for a moment. When you munch down on cruciferous vegetables (kale, cabbage, broccoli, cauliflower, and turnips), your chewing action breaks down their cell walls and a chemical reaction takes place. The plant's sulfur-containing compounds convert into isothiocyanates (ITCs)—a collection of compounds proven to generate powerful immune-boosting and anticancer activity.[2]

One of these compounds is called Nrf2. This amazing factor works with your endothelial cells (the cells that form the lining of your arteries) to prevent adhesion by fat deposits. In other words, it prevents plaque from building up inside your arteries.[3]

It's now wonderfully obvious that, on the third day of Creation, God wrote out the most powerful prescription ever known to human beings to lower the risk of heart disease, our statistically number one killer. How did He do it? He planted a garden.

For more information about how foods affect health and longevity, I highly recommend the books *Super Immunity*, by Joel Fuhrman, MD, and *The Complete Idiot's Guide to Plant-Based Nutrition*, by Julieanna Hever, MS, RD, CPT.[4]

A parting comment: food can be a poison to the systems in our bodies. Food can also be a healer to those systems. The more poisons, the more damage. The more damage, the more symptoms. The more symptoms, the greater need for medications. The more medications, the greater the risk. The greater the risk, the more death.

## Day 4: We've Got Rhythm

What happened on day four of Creation week is as clear as night and day. Actually, it *was* night and day. The night sky became populated with a moon and countless stars, and the day glowed brilliantly under a shimmering sun. What's that got to do with health? Plenty!

We were created to live in harmony with the cycle of light and darkness, day and night. Our bodies create specific hormones for both: serotonin during the day and melatonin at night. These regulate certain bodily functions and help us enjoy both halves of each twenty-four-hour period.

Sunlight provides the catalyst for our bodies' production of that all-important vitamin D. According to Soram Khalsa, MD, in his book, *The Vitamin D Revolution*, "Vitamin D deficiency is now connected to 17 varieties of cancer, along with heart disease, high blood pressure, strokes, autoimmune diseases, diabetes, chronic pain, and osteoporosis."[5]

So, we need sunlight just as much as we need darkness. That's why God created day and night.

There is one problem: we close ourselves off in places where sunlight can't reach us (office cubicles or artificially lit factories) during the day, and at night we bask in the bright glow of our electric lights and television screens. Most of us no longer wake up with the sun, spend the day outdoors, and go to bed when it gets dark. Serotonin/melatonin production keeps getting switched on and off, causing stress to our systems as we motor through sleepy days and energized nights.

What happens when we go against this natural, Creator-ordained rhythm? We put stress on our bodies. We cause our systems to play catch-up—to work when they should be resting and rest when they should be working. The movement of waste material, the triggering of chemical reactions, the ebb and flow of digestion, the energizing of healing cycles, and even the ability to think clearly suffer greatly. A body that's being forced to operate outside its designed parameters is highly prone to disease because the stress greatly weakens its immune system. Add to that a lack of exercise and a poor diet, and you've got yourself a formula for a health disaster. We get sick. We take toxic pills. We get sicker.

Notice I said "healing cycles" in the last paragraph. Don't miss that one. Night, while we're sleeping, is when our bodies turn their attention to healing the wounds of the day. The truth is, our bodies don't ever really "go to sleep." Yes, our thought processes slow down; our digestion comes, almost, to a complete stop; and our oxygen requirements greatly lessen. But our hearts keeps beating, our blood keeps flowing, and our cells keep dividing. Night—while we're sleeping—is when our immune system cranks into high gear, fighting infections and foreign invaders and addressing injuries, using all the resources that are available because they're not off being used to keep us going as they are during the day. The brain also has time to rest and recover so it can continue to function effectively as the command center. All this happens while we drift through the hours of slumber. Take those hours away (or shorten them), and we awake without the benefit of what might have been. Much work is left undone. Now our systems must operate in support of keeping us awake and active. It's easy to see how our tired, overworked bodies can quickly get behind the curve. When that happens, illnesses creep in.

So, enjoy the day, and that all-important exposure to

sunlight, to its fullest. But also enjoy the night by choosing sleep over Leno, keeping the lights low as you head for bed, and making sure your stomach is empty (don't eat anything for four hours before jumping under the covers). That way your body will be ready for the night shift to take over, and you can dream—and heal—under those twinkling stars and the slow-moving moon.

What happens when someone tries to make up for loss of rest? Think of how many medications and stimulants people can avoid just by getting enough rest.

### Day 5: We're Never Alone

Have you ever wondered why God made fish? Birds we can understand. They are beautiful and they sing, filling the forests and glens and our yards with melodies. But fish?

I believe that God created the creatures of the oceans for the very same reason He made birds. Because they're beautiful. Have you ever looked closely at a fish? Amazing design. Extreme colors. Fascinating environment.

Which brings me to an important point about gaining and maintaining optimum health. God never created anything that wasn't important to humanity. I like to believe that fish, birds, and aardvarks, for that matter, exist in part because God didn't want us to ever be lonely. No matter where we wandered, we would have company, even when we went for a swim in the sea. Keep in mind that this was before any living thing attacked any other living thing. This was before such things as fear and predatory impulses separated humanity from the beasts.

On the fifth day of Creation, God began populating this earth with creatures that not only would keep humankind company but also would keep them busy. Animals were created not as primary food sources but as friends, companions, creatures with whom to share God's world. How do you feel when your puppy or kitten greets you at door?

Do you want proof? Have you noticed that the more animals we eat, the sicker we become? In countries with the lowest levels of animal consumption, the residents enjoy the lowest levels of heart disease and cancer. This was brought to light in the book *The China Study*, by epidemiologist Dr. Colin Campbell.[6] Listen to what he says: "The triumph of health lies not in the individual nutrients, but in the whole foods that contain those nutrients: plant-based foods."[7] He also says: "If nutrition were better understood, and prevention and natural treatments were more accepted in the medical community, we would not be pouring so many toxic, potentially lethal drugs into our bodies at the last stage of disease."[8]

I hope you're beginning to see what God had in mind when He spoke animals into existence. Birds and fish fill the sky and waters with life. God loves life. But those same creatures, when consumed by man, can shorten and dull life. God doesn't want that. He has a much higher purpose in mind. Think of this: less animal fat, less cardiovascular disease, less need for a statin drug to lower cholesterol, less risk from a medication.

I know this is hard to read, but I must lovingly speak the truth. For better health we need to eat fewer animals and more plants. As we move in this direction, the chemical benefits to our bodies will become obvious. I tell my patients to eat just enough animal-based foods to keep them happy. And, of course, I hope that in time, very few, if any, animal products will have stayed in their diets. But I also recognize that there is an argument to be made that unhappiness with the foods people are eating may also play a role in their health and must be taken into account. I think this is valid. Each individual is unique, and so we must consider all factors, including whether the food a person is eating is making him or her happy or unhappy. Balance and moderation and loving others without judging them are worth more than words. That is why I say to eat a diet rich in healthful foods and then just enough of the other foods to keep you happy.

On the sixth day, God revealed His hand—and His motivation—in a very dramatic way.

## Day 6: Friends

I wish I could have seen it. Animals everywhere! No cages. No angry growls or death chases. Just animals being friendly to one another, wandering around, exploring their perfect world.

Day six of Creation week has a lot to teach us about

health and how to reduce and even remove our need for pharmaceuticals. In Eden, God's creatures lived in harmony with one another. So, when Adam and Eve came into being, they found themselves in an atmosphere of absolute, perfect love and acceptance.

Love. It's probably the most healing element in life. It calms, brings hope, soothes fears, motivates, endears, sparks creativity, and brings healing to mind and body.

How does love do that? By reducing stress. By turning off the adrenaline pump. By slowing the heartbeat and lowering blood pressure. By relaxing the muscles and centering the thoughts. When you love someone—or are loved—you just feel better.

I believe that's why, on day six, God created more than animals and people. He created an environment that reflected His character of love. Love was reflected in the man caring for the animals and the animals ensuring that the man would never be alone. Love is putting someone or something else's interests above your own.

"The LORD God . . . brought [the animals] to the man to see what he would name them; and whatever the man called each living creature, that was its name" (Genesis 2:19, NIV). God said to Adam and Eve, "Rule over the fish in the sea and the birds in the sky and over every living creature that moves on the ground" (Genesis 1:28, NIV). The word *rule* here means to care for, to be in charge of, to take a special interest in.

Then God said something amazing, something that few

people seem to remember. Listen carefully. God said, "I give you every seed-bearing plant on the face of the whole earth and every tree that has fruit with seed in it. They will be yours for food. And to all the beasts of the earth and all the birds in the sky and all the creatures that move along the ground—everything that has the breath of life in it—I give every green plant for food" (Genesis 1:29-30, NIV).

The Eden diet—the food choices that would assure never-ending longevity—was exactly the same for all creatures. Plants. Fruits. Grains. Nuts. Seeds. Vegetables. The original plan did not include hamburger or chicken nuggets or fish fillets. No pheasant under glass, no beef stew, no pepperoni pizza, no milk, no cream, no eggs. Just plants.

Science demonstrates that the further we force ourselves away from this ideal—the further we wander from it—the less healthy we become. We're changing our diet from what God designed our bodies to optimally handle.

Is it any wonder that there are so many health problems related to consumption? Is it any wonder we're lining up at drugstores to fill endless prescriptions? Does it surprise us that the medications are not fixing the problems and come with inherent risks? Is it any wonder that we're living short and dying long? We are loving less. We've lost track of the very laws that God put in place to keep us healthy! Let's move back on the track. Doing so may help us avoid a dangerous medication.

The very next day, God capped this amazing week with a powerful opportunity to bring healing to both the body and the mind.

## Day 7: Rest

On day seven of Creation week, God instituted the idea of the Sabbath, a time of rest.

During my personal journey of understanding, trying to fathom how we can all learn to live drug free, or at least on fewer drugs, I had no problem seeing the incredible health benefits of staying faithful to naturally occurring circadian rhythms, moving toward a whole-food, plant-based lifestyle, and loving God's creatures. Water intake, air exchange, keeping busy (Adam and Eve were told to "tend" the Garden)—I was totally on board with the science behind each and every one of these health laws. But a day of rest? Why would God create an entire day designed—according to the fourth commandment—for *not* working? And yet, there it is: "You have six days each week for your ordinary work, but the seventh day is a Sabbath day of rest dedicated to the LORD your God. On that day no one in your household may do any work" (Exodus 20:9-10).

Of course, this was before I started seeing patients who were basically keeping most if not all the health laws put in place in Eden but completely ignoring what God had in mind on day seven. Our bodies not only enjoy rest, they *demand* it. We know that. Try staying awake for four days. But apparently, our bodies also demand a *Sabbath* rest, or a full day of rest. This is treatment for a tired mind and body. Here's what I discovered.

Basically, day seven was designed to give us a break

both physically and mentally. For six days we're focused on *working*—on our jobs or professions for paying our bills, our families, our schedules. God designed us to take a break. In this helter-skelter world with its lights-camera-action mentality, are we really getting the rest our bodies need to heal? If you had broken your arm, would you keep throwing fastballs with that arm? No, you would rest and allow it time to heal.

God's design was for us to spend one day a week in rest, both physically and mentally. How might we rest? We might focus on the needs and wants of others. We might attend church to worship God and learn how to better serve our fellow human beings. We might go for a walk in the woods to allow God to inspire us with His handiwork. We might read a good book, one that highlights the life and teaching of someone who has helped humanity. We might visit a friend who is facing some serious challenges. We might get our hands dirty and help someone who can't help him- or herself. We might rest physically by sleeping more. We might spend extra time with friends and family. We might find some extra time to laugh and take care of our own special needs. There are many ways to rest and take a break from our normal routine. I also believe God intended this day of rest to remind us not to get too busy to nurture our relationship with the great Physician. We're to use this time to worship Him and to let Him continue to teach us and lead us in learning to love.

Can you imagine the type of world we'd live in if everyone

did this? Would there be as many wars? Could the crime rate remain high? Could there be a lonely person left anywhere? Would there be as much need for all the prescriptions?

Here's the really amazing part: this Sabbath rest would gladden our hearts as no medicine could. This outward thinking would ease our tension and lower our stress like nothing available at the drugstore. Because that's what love does. That's right. A Sabbath gives us an opportunity to reflect Jesus—the source of all love—to others. Without applying that final health law—the law of love—we're missing an important ingredient necessary for making man and woman whole, allowing us to enjoy optimum health.

**Seven Days, Seven Laws**

There you have it. Seven days of creation. Seven laws of health:

1. Good nutrition—moving toward a whole-food, plant-based diet
2. Exercise—staying active
3. Water—flushing impurities out of the body
4. Sunlight—enjoying the energizing, illness-fighting light of day
5. Air—delivering oxygen to every cell
6. Rest—sleeping and healing all at the same time
7. Sabbath—focusing outside ourselves, learning to love

If you choose not to follow these laws, no police officer will pull you over or knock on your door. The effects may not happen immediately. But stress is put on our systems as we live contrary to the principles in the owner's manual. Just know that something inside you will begin to lose strength, ability, and resistance to disease. Something unseen takes place, the result of which you'll eventually discover in the form of a diagnosis, a pain, a loss of function, or even a loss of life. At the very least, you'll start seeing more and more of your physician . . . and, likely, your local pharmacist. At the pharmacy you might have a prescription filled, and by now, you know the potential dangers.

How did we get in the situation we find ourselves in today? If we understand the past, maybe we can live the present differently so we can change our future. Another voice besides the Creator's spoke in the Garden of Eden. Adam and Eve listened to that other voice, and we're still paying a terrible price for what happened next.

# 12

# THE LAW OF LOVE

*A cheerful heart is good medicine, but a broken spirit*
*saps a person's strength.*
**—PROVERBS 17:22**

HAVE YOU EVER been lied to? I have. I've had individuals look me right in the eye, smile, and speak words that have absolutely no basis in fact. What amazes me is that for some of these people, lying is so incredibly easy.

Psychiatrists tell me that many people who lie don't believe they're doing so. Their fantasy world—the world they've created for themselves, the world in which they choose to live—is so comforting and safe that it has become real to them. So they believe that what they say is the absolute truth, because they desperately need it to be so in order to maintain their illusions.

Others believe that lying makes life easier. They don't

have to support or abide by the truth. And they don't have to do the hard work that the truth requires. Lying is the easy way out—at least for the moment.

Then there's the humorous insight provided by comedian Roseanne Barr in one of her routines: "We women lie to men all the time. It's not because we want to. It's just that it takes so long to explain the truth."

Whatever motivates another person to lie, when we're the victims, we don't like it. We feel cheated and used.

Something else happens to us. We stop trusting those who have lied to us. From that moment on, we don't fully believe what they tell us—even when what they say is actually the truth. We doubt those people, and it may be years before we accept what they say with anything other than a grain of salt.

This brings us to an amazing dichotomy with roots deeply embedded in the past we spoke about in the previous chapter, the time when everything was perfect. We can learn much from the past because it applies not only to the present but also to the future. Within the paradise of Eden, there was initially only truth. But eventually, a lie was told, and choices were made that have affected the health of the world to this day. In the present day, there are still truths and lies. Whom or what are we going to believe?

## Whispers in the Branches

Before I continue, let me share with you what a colleague told me recently: "Jim, if you ended the book at chapter 10, it would be a bestseller by the first medical doctor to fully expose this significant problem. Your simple discussions of solutions would open a new dialogue in medicine and perhaps create a new subspecialty— 'how-to-get-off-medicine-ologists.' But when you bring God into the discussion, you will turn people off. The anti-God people will demean the good things that have been noted and dismiss the book as evangelical propaganda."

I listened and thought about my colleague's words for a time. But how could I ignore what I know to be the truth? Isn't a partial truth still a lie? No, I decided, I would let the reader know about the great Physician and the treatment that changes the heart, the prescription that will give the power to perhaps come off some dangerous medications, and the ultimate healing force in our world and in the universe.

According to the story revealed in Genesis 3, another voice besides God's started to be heard in the Garden. This voice delivered a very different message from what Adam and Eve had been accustomed to hearing from the Creator. You could say that it was the anti-Creator voice, and what it said then continues to reverberate today.

In our mind's eye we can see Adam and Eve in the Garden, perhaps walking along and admiring God's handiwork. At some point, a serpent speaks. I don't know about you, but just *seeing* a snake is enough to send me packing. A *talking* serpent would serve only to double the speed of my exit.

However, for some reason, Adam and Eve felt no such desire to run. Of course, this was before animals became predators. Perhaps talking animals were common in the days after Creation week. Perhaps Adam and Eve had had conversations with this particular creature before. The Bible doesn't say. We do know that nothing in the serpent's appearance, or the fact that it was talking, caused Adam and Eve any discomfort whatsoever. I have to assume that, had I been there, a soft-spoken snake wouldn't have alarmed me, either.

At any rate, the serpent began by asking Eve a question: "Did God really say you must not eat the fruit from any of the trees in the garden?" (Genesis 3:1).

Now Satan—the serpent—was no fool, at least when it came to communicating with humans. His question was designed to allow Eve to correct him, thus placing her—in her mind—on an equal intellectual plane.

"Of course we may eat fruit from the trees in the garden," Eve replied. "It's only the fruit from the tree in the middle of the garden that we are not allowed to eat. God said, 'You must not eat it or even touch it; if you do, you will die'" (Genesis 3:2-3).

Can you see it? Perhaps the serpent nodded slowly, then lowered himself to Eve's eye level. Spreading a smile across his elegant face, he looked Eve in the eye and said, "You won't die! . . . God knows that your eyes will be opened as soon as you eat it, and you will be like God, knowing both good and evil" (Genesis 3:4-5).

Notice something interesting here. Satan blended a lie

(you won't die) with a truth (you'll know both good and evil). Remember that.

You probably know the rest of the story. Eve ate the fruit, gave some to Adam, he ate too, and together they did exactly what God had warned them not to do—they chose to live by a different set of rules. They chose to change the path on which they were traveling, to set themselves up as the final word on what would work and what wouldn't work for their lives.

That path led them right out of Eden and into a world where the serpent—the devil himself—continues to spread his lies to this day. Thankfully, God had a plan in place to remove the eternal separation that Adam's and Eve's decisions caused, but it would take the death of His Son, Jesus, to accomplish it.

The Garden of Eden is long gone. But the lie—those brief words spoken by Satan from the branches of his tree—lives on and on and on. Adam and Eve did die. For millennia people have died. Members of my family and yours have died. Someday, unless Jesus returns first, so will we.

What it comes down to is this: Who was telling the truth? Who offered the correct path? Who knew what was best for our lives? And, in the context of this book, who knew what was best for our health? Is there a universal truth that will help us as we strive to use fewer medications and thus avoid the dangers I have outlined?

The answer to those questions is painfully obvious. God's health plan contained the seven laws we've already identified. There are universal truths in that plan.

In Satan's world,

- Plants are not the preferred source of nutrition.
- Exercise is optional. Instead, enjoy riding in cars, standing on escalators, and spending quality time lounging on easy chairs.
- Water is boring. It's best used as a base ingredient for sodas and alcoholic drinks.
- Sunlight is dangerous. Cover up!
- Air makes a very nice depository for pollution, so keep your windows closed.
- Rest? Who has time? There aren't enough hours in the day. Besides, it's more fun watching late-night TV or hanging out with friends on Facebook. Can't sleep anyway.
- Sabbath rest? Hey, the busier the better. Who needs to connect with their Creator?

On we go, often without realizing that we're moving away from truth, excising God's original health plan from our lives—erasing any remnants of how we were designed to live. We'll be okay. The doctor can fix it. We won't surely die.

### The Missing Ingredient

In the first part of this book, I presented the problem: medicines are killing, and we need to be aware of the risks. By now, I hope, you have also realized that there is an important place for medications. But I want you to ask yourself, *Why am I taking a particular medicine? Is there some other way to change my body's chemistry?* I have offered some simple suggestions, but I want you to look at the past, examine the data for yourself, and find the truth.

Sometimes, however, no matter what we do, we will need medication. There will be suffering. There will be bad outcomes. There may even be the possibility of death. In those instances, where do I go to find hope? There has to be something more than medication. There has to be something more than the health principles given at Creation.

During Adam and Eve's headlong rush to be self-governing and self-sufficient and live outside the protective, nurturing laws God put in place for them, they abandoned one of the most powerful elements of health this planet has ever seen. As a matter of fact, it forms the foundation of all our other actions if we're walking down the path on which God intended for us to journey. I call it the "Law of Love."

The truth is, eating right, living right, doing all the "right" things can take you only so far. Sure, you'll feel better and look better, and maybe even live longer. But will your better, longer life be worth living? By that I mean, Will your life be as joyful and satisfying as it can be?

The answer is no. Because living without love places incredible stress on your body, and we've already discovered some of the far-reaching damage that stress can cause over time. It also does something totally underhanded: it diminishes the good results brought on by doing the "right" things. Let me give you an example.

Suppose you came to my office. After a thorough examination of your cardiovascular system, I determined that you have a dangerous buildup of plaque in your arteries and that this buildup is happening in the one area that's the most dangerous (an arterial branch commonly known as the "widow maker," which would require immediate surgery). I would take care of the immediate danger, of course, and then suggest that you ask yourself why the problem developed in the first place. I would instruct you on what you needed to do to help reverse the condition. This instruction would likely include inviting you to examine all the stressors in your life. Had you been living outside the original plan? Was there a genetic stress that could be modified in some way?

Following my advice faithfully would improve your lot in many profound ways *unless* you were a hateful, vengeful, or angry person. If you despised the world and everyone in it, healing would be greatly curtailed. I could throw endless blood thinners, lifestyle changes, surgeries, cholesterol-lowering drugs, Bible texts, warm fuzzies, and gentle words of encouragement in your direction, and you'd still not experience the full results for which you were hoping. Why? Because feelings of hate, fear, depression, guilt, grief, revenge, and unhappiness have a powerful dulling effect on anything that's supposed to help improve your health. The mind can also change the body's chemistry in profound and as-yet-undiscovered ways. We were designed to think in a certain way.

I like the way King Solomon put it in the Old Testament: "A cheerful heart is good medicine, but a crushed spirit dries up the bones" (Proverbs 17:22, NIV). That old mental-physical connection will get you every time.

Without love in the heart, the heart can't fully heal physically. Similarly, without love in the life, your life remains "sick" and you can never enjoy the wonderful, healing freedom of living in a relationship with God. Love is the missing ingredient, the missing prescription, that so many refuse to accept in their treatment regimens.

That Law of Love permeates all areas of life, from relationships to longevity. It's the ingredient that, like the multitude of phytochemicals in whole-plant foods, enhances all the other ingredients and reactions.

Then why are so many of us experiencing a deep lack of love in our lives? Once again, we must travel back to the Bible to find the answer.

## The Antidote

Do you love God?

Why would I ask such a question in a book exposing the dangers of drugs? As Tina Turner would sing, "What's love got to do with it?"

The answer is simple. Consider this revealing text recorded in the New Testament: "Anyone who does not love does not know God, for God is love" (1 John 4:8). Notice it doesn't say that God loves or God will love or God has loved. It says

God *is* love. He's the embodiment of that particular gift to humanity. This means that whatever He does, His actions are motivated by pure, unadulterated, unfiltered, uncompromising love.

Remember what I said about someone whose life is fueled by hate or anger or a desire for revenge? The stresses generated by these emotions often do more to damage and destroy the human body and mind than all the cigarettes, mixed drinks, and bad habits combined. Stress, whether from unhealthy lifestyle choices or unrelenting, adrenalin-pumping mental stimulation, is an open door for disease.

Here's the clincher: the antidote—the *only, ultimate* antidote—to these destructive elements is love. And the only source of true, pure, healing love is God.

When you top everything off with a strong belief in, and a working relationship with, the Almighty, you'll find that many symptoms—and certainly lifestyle-related diseases—don't stand a chance. Under these circumstances, I'm not talking *good* health, I'm not talking *better* health, I'm talking the *best* health possible.

So, let me ask you again: Do you love God? Because if God is the source of love and you're not connected to that source—for whatever reason—then that *best* treatment will remain out of your reach.

"Yeah, well, God is wonderful and all that," I can hear some people say, "but He is my judge. He's sitting there in heaven just waiting for me to mess up so that someday, in that great judgment to come, He can hurl fire and brimstone down on me. He knows all, sees all, and forgets nothing. If I make mistakes, there will, literally, be hell to pay. And God is behind all that."

Wow! I don't blame you for having a struggle as you try to love that type of God. I don't blame you for not wanting to give yourself over to such a fierce deity. A relationship with that God doesn't sound like love at all. It sounds more like fear, and fear is a major stressor—and we all know what stress does to the human mind or body!

Well, you're in good company. The image of God as a vengeful, raging, angry judge is all too common. As a matter of fact, I believe a misunderstanding of the true character of our heavenly Father is behind much of the spiritual unbelief and mistrust we find in the world today. How can we believe in someone we don't know accurately? How can we love and trust a heavenly being who is just waiting for us to slip up so He can destroy us?

If that line of thinking is standing in the way of your learning to love God and enjoy the far-reaching health benefits of an open and honest relationship with Him, I've got some good news for you! I want you to fall in love with your Creator. Why? Because with that particular relationship operating at full force in your life—with that relationship providing you with the information, motivation, and courage you need in order to live according to the way God designed you to live—you can achieve optimum health and healing. You'll remain less dependent on dangerous and often deadly drugs. Even if there is no way to physically recover from an ailment, there will alway be eternal treatment. God will provide healing in His time.

There are many books written on the subject of God, so I won't attempt to cover every aspect of His beautiful character here, but allow me to focus on just one. Let's look at God through the eyes of someone who knows Him best.

## Choices

I have to admit that as a child, whenever I heard stories about Jesus, I enjoyed every word. But when someone started talking about the Judgment, I got scared and wanted to leave the room. My young mind simply couldn't connect the dots between the grace-filled Savior who healed the sick and the fearful, wrath-filled judge He apparently becomes.

While many people say they're fine with that image of God, insisting that His ways are beyond our comprehension, I just couldn't get comfortable with the concept of a God who seemed—according to what I heard in church—to be saying, "I created you, I love you, I even died for you. But if you don't love me in return, I will kill you."

Once again, I started digging. This is what I discovered.

There was a time in earth's history when the actions of God were not open to human interpretation. They weren't filtered by religious tradition or restraints. For thirty-one years Jesus, the Son of God, lived among us—eating our food, walking our paths, and shivering from the same winter winds that chill us. There were eyewitnesses to His life and times—men who wrote about Him and were amazed by the life-altering power of His message. For one shining moment, God stood completely exposed, illuminated by His own light and expressed by His own words.

It was here I went searching for a God to love.

God asked me to believe in His Son: "God loved the world so much that he gave his one and only Son, so that everyone who believes in him will not perish but have eternal life" (John 3:16). As I reached out to God, He would teach me how to develop a relationship with Him. He would teach me as much as my limited mind could handle in regard to love. He would do the work. He would do the healing. I needed only to accept the gift, God's prescription for life.

Suppose someone says to me, "Dr. Marcum, if you climb up to the top of that cliff and jump off, you're going to fall to the bottom and die," but I climb to the top of the cliff and jump anyway. Sure enough, I fall to the rocks below and am killed instantly. What killed me? What pronounced judgment on me? The power that created gravity? The person who delivered the warning? No. My life ended because I ignored a universal truth: the law of gravity. Another universal truth is this: I was designed to be in a relationship with God. Outside of that relationship there are dangers.

*We* choose whether to jump off the cliff—or not. *We* choose to live in relationship with our Father—or not. *We* choose to live according to His health laws or suffer the chemical changes, the consequences, of not doing so.

I realized that there's salvation riding on the back of God's words as spoken by His Son. There's hope hidden in every syllable. We ignore them at our own peril.

Did the One who spoke those words live by those words? Did He walk the talk?

Jesus came face-to-face with every type of individual. He had the opportunity to judge them openly and severely, and always He demonstrated the part He longs to play in our lives. Let's look at three examples.

## Out on a Limb

As the children's song says, "Zacchaeus was a wee little man." He was small both in stature and in character. As chief tax collector, he went around forcing his fellow countrymen to pay taxes to the despised Romans who forcefully occupied their land. He often collected more than necessary and kept the surplus for himself, which, of course, made him very wealthy. Is it any wonder the Jewish people despised him?

One day, as recorded in Luke 19, Zacchaeus was in Jericho doing what he did best when he heard that Jesus, the famous rabbi who healed the sick, was passing through. Tax-man Zacchaeus wanted to see this popular stranger. But, being a *wee* little man, standing in a curious crowd afforded him a perfect view of only backs and bellies.

Never letting his lack of height interfere with his tall plans, he looked around for a solution and found it towering nearby. Sycamore-fig trees dotted the landscape, and just down the road was a wonderful specimen, complete with sturdy branches and enough leaves to hide his curiosity.

Along comes the Master Teacher surrounded by attentive disciples, a group of recently healed sick people, a gaggle of questioning admirers, and even a few hecklers. Zacchaeus smiled inwardly. He'd found the best seat in the house for the spectacle unfolding below him.

As Jesus reached the tree, He stopped.

When I was young, I always smiled at this point in the story. *Now Zacchaeus is going to get it*, I'd think. *That crook has come face-to-face with the God of the universe. Stand back, everyone!*

Here's the way I pictured it: slowly, with a smile lighting His face, Jesus looked up—right at Zacchaeus. The tax man may have grinned self-consciously, suddenly wishing he were much smaller than he already was.

"Zacchaeus," the Master Teacher called, "come down immediately. I must stay at your house today."

In stunned wonder, the short man made the long journey from his tree limb to the ground. "You want to come to *my* house?" he asked.

Christ nodded.

"This way," Zacchaeus stammered, pointing down the road. "Just . . . follow me."

Later, after Zacchaeus and Jesus had spent some time together, an incredible thing happened to the little man. He grew up. Not in height, but in character. He said to Jesus, "I will give half my wealth to the poor, Lord, and if I have cheated people on their taxes, I will give them back four times as much!" (Luke 19:8).

Zacchaeus the crooked tax collector met Jesus the Judge face-to-face. And Jesus' "sentence" was "Invite me to your home." Zacchaeus believed in the true God, and he was changed by the power of the relationship.

## Undercover Sinner

One day, in early morning, Jesus was spending time teaching at the Temple in Jerusalem when a group of men brought a woman to Jesus and put her in front of the crowd. "'Teacher,' they said to Jesus, 'this woman was caught in the act of adultery. The law of Moses says to stone her. What do you say?'" (John 8:4-5).

*Yes, Jesus,* I thought to myself, *what do you say? She's a home wrecker, a wicked woman, a sinner.*

Jesus told the men, "All right, but let the one who has never sinned throw the first stone!" (v. 7). Then He bent down and started writing in the dust with His finger. I have no idea what He wrote, but the men must have seen something that made them decide they were late for an appointment elsewhere.

Soon, only Jesus and the accused remained—sinner and judge standing face-to-face.

Jesus asked her, "Where are your accusers? Didn't even one of them condemn you?" (v. 10).

The woman, sensing that this confrontation was going to

turn out quite different from what she'd expected, answered, "No, Lord" (v. 11).

The next words out of Jesus' mouth, combined with the story of Zacchaeus, changed the way I looked at Christ and the future. Jesus may have gazed intently into the woman's eyes as He said, "Neither do I. Go and sin no more" (v. 11). He loved her. He forgave her. That relationship once again gave power to the believer. Her life was changed. It was that simple.

## Hanging in the Balance

Finally, my search for truth took me to a very dark place—a hilltop just outside the walls of Jerusalem where I found Christ hanging in agony on a Roman cross. On each side of Him, impaled on their own instruments of torture, were two sinners—thieves whose lives had been filled with violence and lawlessness.

One cursed the dying Savior with these mocking words: "So you're the Messiah, are you? Prove it by saving yourself—and us, too, while you're at it!" (Luke 23:39).

The other thief turned to his fellow criminal and groaned through his pain, "Don't you fear God even when you have been sentenced to die? We deserve to die for our crimes, but this man hasn't done anything wrong" (vv. 40-41).

Then, looking over at the Savior, he added, "Jesus, remember me when you come into your Kingdom" (v. 42).

Jesus answered, "I assure you, today you will be with me in paradise" (v. 43).

Someday I'm going to stand beside the tax man, the adulterous woman, and the thief who believed on the cross and look into the face of the one who judged us all worthy of salvation because of His Son's sacrifice. We'll walk the streets of heaven because we believed Jesus' words and felt the eternal touch of God's judgment of love. This is the ultimate healing. This relationship with God will give you the power to find truth and to change your life. This is the "something more" I wanted to tell you about. These truths from the past can be used to change the present and prepare us for the future.

### A New Relationship

"Come to me, all of you who are weary and carry heavy burdens, and I will give you rest" (Matthew 11:28). Jesus said this. *Come to me. Worship me. Develop a relationship with me. You might be carrying heavy burdens, stressed by the world or your genetics. But when you come to me, a gift is waiting. I will give you peace. I will give you healing. I will change the chemistry of your life.*

If you want to live your life unburdened by the dangerous intrusion of modern medicines, if you want to build and maintain optimum health, if you want to enjoy the healing presence of God in your life, it's time to start forming a new relationship with your Creator and live by the healing truth of His words.

How do you do that? First, you begin by accepting God's free gift and asking Him to teach you how to have a relationship with Him. Talk to Him. Listen to Him through His Word, the Bible, through nature, and through His ambassadors.

As you do this, He will continue to reveal Himself to you. You will learn to love God—the real God, the God embodied by Jesus. As your heart and mind become flooded with His teaching and presence, many of the stresses caused by the world will begin to fall away. You will be changed. The hate, the feelings of revenge, the anger over life's multitude of unfair events and unkind acts will lose their grip on you. You'll begin to realize that you, yes *you*, are loved. And from this new foundation, you'll feel compelled to reach out and love others. Your chemistry will change. Along with the health laws outlined by God in Genesis, that missing and powerful Law of Love will become a reality in your life, and you'll find that many of the aches and pains, the concerns that cloud your thinking, and the feelings of worthlessness you often experience will slowly fade away.

It all comes down to choices. Medicines can kill. But God can heal. Within His health laws, including love, which governs the universe, we find new life, both here and in the world to come.

Jesus said, "It is my Father's will that all who see his Son and believe in him should have eternal life" (John 6:40). That eternal life, that life filled with joy and healing—free from many of the dangers of modern medicine and deadly drugs—can begin today. The choice is yours. This is the "something more" I hope you will make a part of your life.

# Appendix A:
# Drugs Withdrawn
# from the Market

THE FOLLOWING is a partial list of drugs withdrawn from the market and a timeline of those withdrawals.

- Thalidomide: withdrawn from various markets during the 1950s and early 1960s due to the risk of severe birth defects. More recently used as an anticancer drug.
- Lysergic acid diethylamide (LSD): withdrawn in the 1950s and 1960s. Originally marketed as a psychiatric medication, it was sometimes used recreationally.
- Diethylstilbestrol: withdrawn in the 1970s also due to the risk of birth defects.

- Phenformin and buformin: withdrawn in 1978 because of risk of lactic acidosis, the buildup of lactic acid in the bloodstream faster than the body can remove it.
- Ticrynafen: withdrawn in 1982 due to a high risk of hepatitis.
- Zimelidine: withdrawn worldwide in 1983 due to a heightened risk of Guillain-Barré syndrome.
- Phenacetin: withdrawn in 1983 because of risk of cancer and kidney disease.
- Methaqualone: withdrawn in 1984 due to the risk of addiction and overdose.
- Nomifensine: withdrawn in 1986 because of the risk of hemolytic anemia.
- Triazolam (trade name Halcion): withdrawn in the United Kingdom in 1991 because of risk of psychiatric adverse reactions. It is still available in the US.
- Temafloxacin (trade name Omniflox): withdrawn in 1992 because of allergic reactions and cases of hemolytic anemia.
- Flosequinan: withdrawn in 1993 due to an increased risk of abnormal heart rhythms as well as increased hospitalizations and death.
- Alpidem: withdrawn in 1996 because of rare but serious hepatotoxicity (liver damage).
- Chlormezanone: withdrawn in 1996 due to rare but serious cases of toxic shedding of the top layer of skin (epidermal necrolysis).

- Fen-Phen: withdrawn in 1997 due to risk of heart-valve disorder.
- Tolrestat: withdrawn in 1997 due to risk of severe hepatotoxicity (liver damage).
- Dexfenfluramine (trade name Redux): withdrawn in 1997 because of the risk of many adverse reactions, including abnormal heart rhythms and blood pressure problems.
- Fenfluramine (trade name Pondimin): withdrawn in 1997, after 290 months on the market, due to the risk of heart-valve disease.
- Terfenadine (trade names Seldane or Triludan): withdrawn in 1998 due to the risk of cardiac arrhythmias.
- Mibefradil (trade name Posicor): withdrawn in 1998 due to dangerous interactions with other drugs.
- Etretinate: withdrawn in 1990s due to the risk of birth defects.
- Tolcapone (trade name Tasmar): withdrawn in 1998 due to a risk of hepatotoxicity (liver damage).
- Temazepam (trade name Restoril): withdrawn in 1999 in Sweden and Norway due to recreational use and abuse and a high rate of overdose deaths. It is still available in the United States.
- Astemizole (trade name Hismanal): withdrawn in 1999 due to interactions with other drugs that caused heart arrhythmias.

- Levamisole (trade name Ergamisol): withdrawn in 1999 because of a link to serious blood disease.
- Bromfenac (trade name Duract): withdrawn in 1999 because of risk of liver failure.
- Grepafloxacin (trade name Raxar): withdrawn in 2000 because of risk of heart arrhythmias.
- Trogalitazone (trade name Rezulin): withdrawn in 2000 due to the risk of hepatotoxicity (liver damage); superseded by pioglitazone and rosiglitazone.
- Alosetron (trade name Lotronex): withdrawn in 2000 because of risk of fatal complications of constipation; reintroduced on a limited basis in 2002.
- Cisapride (trade name Propulsid): withdrawn in 2000 due to risk of irregular heart rhythms.
- Amineptine (trade name Survector): withdrawn in 2000 due to the risk of liver damage.
- Phenylpropanolamine: withdrawn in 2000 due to the high risk of stroke in women under fifty when taken at high doses for purposes of weight loss.
- Trovafloxacin (trade name Trovan): withdrawn in 2001 due to risk of liver damage.
- Cerivastatin (trade name Baycol): withdrawn in 2001 due to risk of rhabdomyolysis, a breakdown of muscle fiber that leads to the release of those fiber contents into the bloodstream and subsequent kidney damage.
- Rapacuronium bromide (trade name Raplon): withdrawn in 2001 because it could cause fatal bronchospasms.

- Rofecoxib (trade name Vioxx): withdrawn in 2004 due to a risk of myocardial infarction (heart attack).
- Co-proxamol (trade name Distalgesic): withdrawn in 2004 in the United Kingdom due to a high incidence of accidental deaths related to its use.
- Hydromorphone extended release (trade name Palladone): withdrawn in 2005 because of a high risk of accidental overdose when used with alcohol.
- Thioridazine (trade name Mellaril): withdrawn in 2005 in Canada because of the risk of potentially fatal heart damage.
- Pemoline (trade name Cylert): withdrawn in 2005 because it could cause liver damage or liver failure.
- Natalizumab (trade name Tysabri): voluntarily withdrawn in 2005–2006 because of risk of progressive multifocal leukoencephalopathy, a severe neurological disease. Returned to the market in 2006.
- Ximelagatran (trade name Exanta): withdrawn in 2006 because it could cause liver damage.
- Pergolide (trade name Permax): voluntarily withdrawn in 2007 in the US due to risk of heart-valve damage. Still available elsewhere.
- Tegaserod (trade name Zelnorm): withdrawn in 2007 because it could cause heart attack and stroke.
- Aprotinin (trade name Trasylol): withdrawn in 2007 because use carried a risk of complications such as kidney failure, heart failure, heart attack, or death.

- Inhaled insulin (trade name Exubera): withdrawn in 2007 due to doubts over long-term safety.
- Lumiracoxib (trade name Prexige): withdrawn in 2007–2008 due to serious side effects, including liver damage.
- Rimonabant (trade name Acomplia): withdrawn in 2008 because it could cause severe depression and suicide.
- Efalizumab (trade name Raptiva): withdrawn in 2009 because of increased risk of progressive multifocal leukoencephalopathy, a fatal brain infection.
- Sibutramine (trade name Meridia): withdrawn in 2010 due to increased risk of cardiovascular problems.
- Gemtuzumab ozogamicin (trade name Mylotarg): withdrawn in 2010 due to increased risk of veno-occlusive disease (i.e., blockage of tiny veins).
- Rosiglitazone (trade name Avandia): withdrawn in 2010 in Europe because of increased rates of heart attacks and death. Still available in the United States.

# Appendix B: Food and Drug Administration (FDA) Medication Classifications

**Schedule 1 Medications:** The use of these substances—which include lysergic acid diethylamide (LSD), peyote, heroin, and marijuana—is illegal. Some states have legalized the use of marijuana for medicinal purposes.

**Schedule 2 Medications:** Narcotics are in this class. These substances are prone to cause addiction and abuse. Misuse of the medications in this class is life threatening. Doctors may legally prescribe these risky medications with special precautions.

**Schedule 3 Medications:** These include milder sleeping pills, pain medications, and tranquilizers. The substances in this class can be abused, but the potential for abuse is less likely than for schedule 2 medications.

**Schedule 4 Medications:** These medications include blood pressure pills, antibiotics, and other medicines that require specific doses and should be used only under a doctor's supervision. Abuse is unlikely, but the medications might be hazardous if use is unsupervised.

**Schedule 5 Medications:** These are over-the-counter medicines. Ibuprofen, acetaminophen, aspirin, and vitamins fall into this class. Their use does not require a doctor's supervision, but they can still have risks.

As this book has illustrated, all the medicines in these classes can kill given the right set of circumstances.

# Appendix C:
# How a Medication Gets to Market

THREE HUNDRED YEARS AGO, if physicians did not use leeches to pull blood from feverish patients, they were not considered good doctors. For most of the history of the world, medicine men and families have been practicing the art of healing without regulation or oversight. Upton Sinclair's book *The Jungle*, written in the early 1900s, exposed the issue of contaminated food and influenced a nation to become more vigilant about health concerns. In 1906, the Pure Food and Drug Act was passed. This led to the establishment of what eventually became known as the Food and Drug Administration (FDA). The FDA had the authority to regulate and control the flow of drugs. It required a manufacturer to submit evidence that the medication or other product was safe.

Subsequent legislation in 1912 prohibited false and fraudulent claims. Remember the old movies with the cure-all elixirs? In 1938, the Food, Drug, and Cosmetic Act was passed. In 1962, the Kefauver-Harris Amendment required drug manufacturers not only to prove that each drug they produced was safe but also to provide evidence from the results of scientific studies for the drug's effectiveness. The Fair Packaging and Labeling Act, passed in 1966, required that products "be honestly and informatively labeled."[1] This was the forerunner to the patient package inserts we see today. In 1971, the Drug Quality Reporting System was established to track the reporting of adverse events.

The FDA's Center for Drug Evaluation and Research has a protocol for evaluating new medications. After a pharmaceutical company develops and synthesizes a medication with potential, it submits a New Drug Application. The center requires the medication to be safety tested on two different animal species. In this stage, scientists learn the dosages needed to achieve both beneficial and toxic effects, as well as how the drug is absorbed and eliminated by the body. The preclinical trial gains this information on the new medication and determines its safety. If the trial goes well, a Phase I trial begins. This is a human trial in which twenty to eighty volunteers are given the medication to test how the body

---

[1] *FDA Consumer Magazine* (January–February 2006).

metabolizes the medicine, how the medicine actually works in the body, and any side effects. The goal is to evaluate the drug in human bodies. Usually the members of this study group are healthy individuals. If there are no significant problems discovered in Phase I testing, a Phase II trial begins. In this phase several hundred patients are placed in a controlled clinical trial. This phase evaluates the medication's effectiveness for a given disease and also tests for adverse reactions.

If the results of the Phase II trials do not eliminate a medication, the medication moves to a Phase III trial. This study includes hundreds to several thousand patients. The more patients and diverse groups studied at this stage, the better. If the results of Phase III testing are positive, the medication is approved for use, and marketing to millions begins. The manufacturer pays for the research, development, and clinical trials. This is a costly process.

The approval process involves billions of dollars and takes years to complete. Chemists, researchers, lawyers, politicians, marketers, and pharmaceutical representatives are some of the professionals involved in the process.

Next, millions of patients use the medication. Physicians are encouraged to report adverse reactions and side effects not previously discovered in earlier testing. If adverse reports are significant, the FDA requires the manufacturer to place a "black-box" warning on either the medication's label or in the literature related to the drug. At times, a recall of the medication is ordered. Unfortunately, whenever millions of dollars are involved, there is the chance of unethical behavior during the trials prior to bringing a medication to the market. Politics, as you might imagine, can be involved, and the Internet is loaded with information on the topic. For the purpose of this book, be aware that we do not live in a perfect world. Sometimes dangerous warnings regarding the safety of a medication are unheeded for the sake of the almighty dollar.

# Appendix D: Most-Prescribed Medications in 2010[1]

1. hydrocodone—for chronic pain: 131.2 million prescriptions in 2010; 128.2 million prescriptions in 2009

2. simvastatin (brand name Zocor)—for high cholesterol (36 million Americans have high cholesterol levels): 94.1 million prescriptions in 2010; 83.8 million prescriptions in 2009

3. lisinopril—for high blood pressure: 87.4 million prescriptions in 2010; 82.8 million prescriptions in 2009

4. levothyroxine sodium (brand name Synthroid)—for low thyroid levels: 70.5 million prescriptions in 2010; 66 million prescriptions in 2009

[1] "The Use of Medicines in the United States: Review of 2010," Report by the IMS Institute for Healthcare Informatics, 33. Also available at www.imshealth.com/imshealth/Global/Content/IMS%20Institute/Documents/IHII_UseOfMed_report%20.pdf. Accessed October 4, 2012.

5. amlodipine besylate (brand name Norvasc)—for lowering blood pressure (high blood pressure affects 2 out of 3 people over sixty): 57.2 million prescriptions in 2010; 51.3 million prescriptions in 2009

6. omeprazole (brand names Prilosec, Omesec)—for blocking acid production in the stomach: 53.4 million prescriptions in 2010; 45.4 million prescriptions in 2009

7. azithromycin—for bacterial infections: 52.6 million prescriptions in 2010; 53.8 million prescriptions in 2009

8. amoxicillin—another antibiotic for bacterial infections such as strep throat: 52.3 million prescriptions in 2010; 52.4 million prescriptions in 2009

9. metformin HCL (brand names Fortamet, Glucophage)—for diabetes, 48.3 million prescriptions in 2010; 44.3 million prescriptions in 2009. These numbers are soaring, with 25.8 million people suffering from diabetes.

10. HCTZ (hydrochlorothiazide)—for high blood pressure: 47.8 million prescriptions in 2010; 47.9 million prescriptions in 2009

Total prescriptions written each year in America alone: approximately 3 billion, according to the US Food and Drug Administration Safe Use Initiative Fact Sheet.[2]

---

[2] Available at www.fda.gov/Drugs/DrugSafety/ucm188760.htm, accessed September 26, 2012.

# Notes

## CHAPTER 2. IT COULD HAPPEN TO YOU

1. Rainu Kaushal, MD, MPH et al, "Medication Errors and Adverse Drug Events in Pediatric Inpatients," *Journal of the American Medical Association* 285, no. 16 (April 25, 2001): 2114–2120.

## CHAPTER 3. MEDICAL MISTAKES

1. Gary Null, PhD, et al, "Death by Medicine," *Life Extension* (March 2004). www.lef.org/magazine/mag2004/mar2004_awsi_death_02. Accessed August 23, 2012.
2. Null et al, "Death by Medicine."
3. Null et al, "Death by Medicine."
4. Lucien Leape, MD, "Error in Medicine," *Journal of the American Medical Association* 272, no. 23 (December 21, 1994): 1851–57.
5. David Barboza, "2,000 Arrested in China in Counterfeit Drug Crackdown," *New York Times* (August 5, 2012): A6. Also available at www.nytimes .com/2012/08/06/world/asia/2000-arrested-in-china-in-crackdown-on -counterfeit-drugs.html?_r=0. Accessed September 4, 2012.

6. "FDA Has Conducted More Foreign Inspections and Begun to Improve Its Information on Foreign Establishments, but More Progress Is Needed," report from the US Government Accountability Office, September 30, 2010. Available at www.gao.gov/products/GAO-10-961. Accessed August 24, 2012.

7. David P. Phillips, PhD, et al, "A Spike in Fatal Medication Errors at the Beginning of Each Month," *Pharmacotherapy* 25, no. 1 (2005): 1.

8. David P. Phillips, PhD, and Gwendolyn E. C. Barker, BA, "A July Spike in Fatal Medication Errors: A Possible Effect of New Medical Residents," *Journal of General Internal Medicine* (May 29, 2010): 774–79.

9. Susanna Bedell, MD, et al, "Discrepancies in the Use of Medications: Their Extent and Predictors in an Outpatient Practice," *Archives of Internal Medicine* (July 24, 2000): 2130.

10. Sunil Kripalani, MD, et al, "Effect of a Pharmacist Intervention on Clinically Important Medication Errors after Hospital Discharge: A Randomized Trial," *Annals of Internal Medicine* 157, no. 1 (July 3, 2012): 1–10.

11. "Adult Literacy in America," report from the US Department of Education Office of Education Research and Improvement, 3rd ed. (April 2002): xvii. Available at http://nces.ed.gov/pubs93/93275.pdf. Accessed August 24, 2012.

12. "The Literacy Problem," www.hsph.harvard.edu/healthliteracy/files/doakchap1-4.pdf. Accessed August 24, 2012.

13. Julie A. Gazmararian et al, "Health Literacy and Knowledge of Chronic Disease," *Patient Education and Counseling* 51, no. 3 (November 2003): 267–75. Available at www.pec-journal.com/article/S0738-3991(02)00239-2/abstract. Accessed August 24, 2012.

## CHAPTER 4. ADVERSE REACTIONS AND INSUFFICIENT RESEARCH

1. Alfred I. Neugut, MD, PhD; Anita T. Ghatak, MPH; and Rachel L. Miller, MD, "Anaphylaxis in the United States: An Investigation into Its Epidemiology," *Archives of Internal Medicine* 161, no. 1 (January 2001). Available at http://archinte.jamanetwork.com/article.aspx?articleid=646961. Accessed August 27, 2012.

2. Neugut, Ghatak, and Miller, "Anaphylaxis in the United States."

3. Geneva, Switzerland: World Health Organization, 1969. "International Drug Monitoring: The Role of Hospital"(Technical report series no. 425).

4. T. R. Einarson, "Drug-Related Hospital Admissions," *Annals of Pharmacotherapy* 27, no. 7/8 (July/August 1993): 832–40. Also available at www.theannals.com/content/27/7/832.abstract. Accessed August 27, 2012.

5. T. A. Brennan et al, "Incidence of Adverse Events and Negligence in Hospitalized Patients. Results of the Harvard Medical Practice Study I," *New England Journal of Medicine* (February 7, 1991): 370–76.

6. David C. Classen, MD, et al, "Adverse Drug Events in Hospitalized Patients," *Journal of the American Medical Association* 277, no. 4 (January 22, 1997). Available at http://jama.jamanetwork.com/article .aspx?articleid=413536. Accessed August 27, 2012.

7. Mukeshkumar B. Vora et al, "Adverse Drug Reactions in Inpatients of Internal Medicine Wards at a Tertiary Care Hospital: A Prospective Cohort Study," *Journal of Pharmacology and Pharmacotherapeutics* 2, no. 1 (January–March 2011): 21–25. Also available at www.ncbi.nlm.nih.gov /pmc/articles/PMC3117564. Accessed September 5, 2012.

8. "Risks and Benefits of Estrogen plus Progestin in Healthy Postmenopausal Women," *Journal of the American Medical Association*, 288, no. 3 (July 17, 2002): 321–33. Also available at http://jama.jamanetwork.com/article. aspx?articleid=195120. Accessed August 27, 2012.

9. Valerie Beral, "Breast Cancer and Hormone-Replacement Therapy in the Million Women Study," *Lancet* (August 9, 2003): 419–27. Also available at www.ncbi.nlm.nih.gov/pubmed/12927427. Accessed August 27, 2012.

10. K. A. Schulman et al, "Economic Analysis of Conventional-Dose Chemotherapy Compared with High-Dose Chemotherapy plus Autologous Hematopoietic Stem-Cell Transplantation for Metastatic Breast Cancer," *Bone Marrow Transplantation*, 31 (2003): 205–10. Also available at www.nature.com/bmt/journal/v31/n3/abs/1703795a.html. Accessed August 27, 2012.

11. Martin H. Teicher et al, "Emergence of Intense Suicidal Preoccupation during Fluoxetine Treatment," *American Journal of Psychiatry*, 147 (February 1990), 207–10.

12. Thomas H. Maugh II, "Banned Report on Vioxx Published," *Los Angeles Times* (January 25, 2005).

13. David Graham et al, "Risk of Acute Myocardial Infarction and Sudden Cardiac Death in Patients Treated with Cyclo-oxygenase 2 Selective and Non-selective Non-steroidal Anti-inflammatory Drugs: Nested Control Study," *Lancet*, 365 (February 5, 2005): 475–81. Also available at http://www.thelancet.com/journals/lancet/article/PIIS0140-6736%2805 %2917864-7/abstract. Accessed September 6, 2012.

14. Duff Wilson, "Merck to Pay $950 Million Over Vioxx," *New York Times* (November 22, 2011).

15. Deposition of Dr. Raymond Pogge (July 26, 1976), Mekdeci vs. Merrell National Laboratories, case #77-255 Ore-Civ-Y, 50-51.

16. Physicians Committee for Responsible Medicine, "Birth Defect Statistics," www.pcrm.org/search/?cid=2785. Accessed August 27, 2012.

17. E. B. Schwarz et al, "Frequency of Birth Control Services with Prescriptions for Unsafe Drugs During Pregnancy," *Annals of Internal Medicine* 147, no. 6 (September 18, 2007): 1–38. Also available at http://annals.org/article .aspx?articleid=736681. Accessed August 27, 2012.

18. Thomas Delate, PhD et al, "Trends in the Use of Antidepressants in a National Sample of Commercially Insured Pediatric Patients, 1998–2002," *Psychiatric Services* 55, no. 4 (April 2004): 387–91. Also available at http://ps.psychiatryonline.org/data/Journals/PSS/3612/387.pdf. Accessed September 5, 2012.

19. Cited in Bob Murray, PhD, and Alicia Fortenberry, "Pill-Popping Pre-Schoolers," April 3, 2004, www.upliftprogram.com/h_depression .html#h77. Accessed October 24, 2112.

20. Anne M. Larson et al, "Acetaminophen-induced Acute Liver Failure: Results of a United States Multicenter Prospective Study," *Hepatology* 42, no. 6 (December 2005): 1364–72.

21. David Willman, "How a New Policy Led to Seven Deadly Drugs," *Los Angeles Times* (December 20, 2000). Also available at www.latimes.com /news/nationworld/nation/la-122001fda,0,3054990.story. Accessed September 5, 2012.

## CHAPTER 5. MISUSE OF MEDICATIONS

1. Leonard Paulozzi, MD, et al, "CDC Grand Rounds: Prescription Drug Overdoses—a U.S. Epidemic," Centers for Disease Control and Prevention (January 13, 2012): 10–13. Also available at www.cdc.gov/mmwr/preview /mmwrhtml/mm6101a3.htm. Accessed August 28, 2012.

2. Shari Roan, "Drug Poisoning Deaths Continue Tragic Climb," *Los Angeles Times* (December 20, 2011). Available at http://articles.latimes.com /2011/dec/20/news/la-heb-poisoning-deaths-20111220. Accessed August 28, 2012.

3. Genevra Pittman, "1 in 8 Teens Misuses Prescription Painkillers," Reuters News Service (May 8, 2012). Available at www.msnbc.msn.com/id /47329424/ns/health-childrens_health/t/teens-misuses-prescription -painkillers. Accessed August 28, 2012.

4. Tom Blackwell, "Prozac Defense Stands in Manitoba Teen's Murder Case," *National Post* (December 7, 2011). Also available at http://news .nationalpost.com/2011/12/07/prozac-defence-stands-in-manitoba-teens -murder-case. Accessed August 28, 2012.

5. Qiuping Gu, MD, et al, "Prescription Drug Use Continues to Increase: U.S. Prescription Drug Data for 2007–2008," *NCHS Brief* 42 (September

2010). Available at www.cdc.gov/nchs/data/databriefs/db42.htm. Accessed September 5, 2012.

6. Joseph G. Cote, "Prescription Painkillers Emerging as Leading Threat among Drugs," NashuaTelegraph.com (June 24, 2012).

7. Nora D. Volkow, MD, Introduction to "Prescription Drugs: Abuse and Addiction," National Institute on Drug Abuse Research Report Series (October 2011). Also available at http://m.drugabuse.gov/sites/default /files/rrprescription.pdf. Accessed August 28, 2012.

8. Nate Rau, "Tennessee Lawmakers Tighten Regulations for Prescription Pain Pills," *The Tennessean* (January 30, 2012).

9. Aron J. Hall et al, "Patterns of Abuse among Unintentional Pharmaceutical Overdose Facilities," *Journal of the American Medical Association* 300, no. 22 (December 10, 2008).

10. Hall et al, "Patterns of Abuse."

## CHAPTER 6. SLOW KILL AND DEADLY COMBINATIONS

1. Neal Barnard, MD, *Breaking the Food Seduction* (New York: St. Martin's Griffin, 2004), 2.

2. Erick Smith, "Autopsy: Alabama OL Aaron Douglas Died of 'Multiple Drug Toxicity," *USA Today*, June 28, 2011. Also available at http://content .usatoday.com/communities/campusrivalry/post/2011/06/alabama-aaron -douglas-autopsy-report-drugs/1. Accessed October 1, 2012.

3. Erick Smith, "Oklahoma Linebacker Austin Box Dead at the Age of 22," *USA Today*, May 19, 2011. Also available at http://content.usatoday.com /communities/campusrivalry/post/2011/05/oklahoma-linebacker-austin -box-dead/1. Accessed October 1, 2012.

4. Allen J. Frances, MD, "Polypharmacy, PTSD, and Accidental Death from Prescription Medication," *Psychology Today* (February 13, 2011).

5. Melonie Herron, PhD, "Deaths: Leading Causes for 2007," *National Vital Statistics Reports* 59, no. 8 (August 26, 2011): Table C, page 9. Also available at www.cdc.gov/nchs/data/nvsr/nvsr59/nvsr59_08.pdf. Accessed October 1, 2012.

6. W. A. Eggar, "Antibiotic Resistance: Unnatural Selection in the Office and on the Farm," *Wisconsin Medical Journal* (August 2002).

7. R. Rabin, "Caution about Overuse of Antibiotics," *Newsday* (September 18, 2003). Cited in Gary Null, PhD, "Death by Medicine," www.whale .to/a/null9.html#The_Problem_with_Antibiotics. Accessed August 29, 2012.

8. D. R. Nash et al, "Antibiotic Prescribing by Primary Care Physicians for Children with Upper Respiratory Infections," *Pediatric Adolescent Medicine*

156, no. 11 (November 2002): 1114–19. Also available at www.ncbi.nlm
.nih.gov/pubmed/12413339.

9. John M. Hickner, MD, et al, "Principles of Appropriate Antibiotic Use
for Acute Rhinosinusitis in Adults," *Annals of Internal Medicine* 134, no. 6
(March 20, 2001): 498–505.

10. R. Mangione-Smith et al, "The Relationship between Perceived Parental
Expectations and Pediatrician Antimicrobial Prescribing Behavior,"
*Pediatrics* 103 (1999): 711–18.

11. J. G. Scott et al, "Antibiotic Use in Upper Respiratory Infections and the
Ways Patients Pressure Physicians for a Prescription," *Journal of Family
Practice* 50, no. 10 (2001): 853–58.

12. A. Mark Fendrick et al, "The Economic Burden of Non-Influenza-Related
Viral Respiratory Tract Infection in the United States," *Archives of Internal
Medicine* 163, no. 4 (2003): 487–94.

13. Robert A. Weinstein, "Nosocomial Infection Update," *Emerging Infectious
Diseases (special update)* 4, no. 3 (July–September, 1998): 416–19. Also
available at wwwnc.cdc.gov/eid/article/4/3/pdfs/98-0320.pdf. Accessed
September 5, 2012.

## CHAPTER 7. OVER-THE-COUNTER MEDICATIONS

1. "OTC Medicines/Dietary Supplements Facts and Figures," Consumer
Healthcare Products Association, www.chpa-info.org/pressroom/OTC
_FactsFigures.aspx. Accessed August 29, 2012.

2. "OTC Medicines/Dietary Supplements Facts and Figures," CHPA.

3. Jarrett Murphy, "Ephedra Tied to Pitcher's Death," *CBS Evening News*,
February 11, 2009. Available at www.cbsnews.com/2100-18563_162
-540848.html. Accessed August 29, 2012.

4. Gurley, B. J., et al, "Ephedrine Pharmacokinetics after the Ingestion
of Nutritional Supplements Containing Ephedra Sinica (Ma Huang),"
*Therapeutic Drug Monitoring* 4 (August 20, 1998): 439–45.

5. Anne-Marie O'Neill, "Fatal Choice," *People* 52, no. 4 (August 2, 1999).
Available at www.people.com/people/archive/article/0,,20128865,00.html.
Accessed August 29, 2012.

6. Ralph I. Horowitz, MD, et al, "Phenylpropanolamine and Risk of
Hemorrhagic Stroke: Final Report of the Hemorrhagic Stroke Project,"
May 10, 2000. Available at www.fda.gov/ohrms/dockets/ac/00/backgrd
/3647b1_tab19.doc. Accessed August 29, 2012.

7. B. K. Logan et al, "Five Deaths Resulting from Abuse of Dextromethorphan
Sold over the Internet," *Journal of the Annals of Toxicology* 33, no. 2 (March

2009): 99–103. Available at www.ncbi.nlm.nih.gov/pubmed/19239735. Accessed September 6, 2012.

8. Pediatric Toxicology Committee and Data Committee, National Association of Medical Examiners, "Infant Deaths Associated with Cough and Cold Medications—Two States, 2005," *Morbidity and Mortality Weekly Report* 56, no. 1 (January 12, 2007): 1–4. Available at www.cdc.gov/mmwr /preview/mmwrhtml/mm560121.htm. Accessed September 6, 2012.

9. Teri Robert, "Teenager Dies from Acetaminophen Overdose" (September 7, 2006). Available at http://headaches.about.com/cs/medicationsusage /a/acet_death.htm. Accessed August 29, 2012.

10. Anne M. Larson et al, "Acetaminophen-Induced Acute Liver Failure," *Hepatology* 42, no. 6 (2005): 1368.

**PART 2. THE SOLUTION**

1. Joel J. Nobel, MD, "Technology Assessment Policy: Top Down or Bottom Up?," *Journal of Health Policy* 9, no. 3 (1998): 337–39.

**CHAPTER 8. SOMETIMES YOU NEED TO THINK**

1. Qiuping Gu, MD, et al, "Prescription Drug Use Continues to Increase: U.S. Prescription Drug Data for 2007–2008," *NCHS Brief* 42 (September 2010). Available at www.cdc.gov/nchs/data/databriefs/db42.htm. Accessed August 29, 2012.

**CHAPTER 10. LET'S GET PRACTICAL, PART 2**

1. Jennifer Welsh, "Why Laughter May Be the Best Pain Medicine," *Scientific American* (September 14, 2011). Also available at www.scientificamerican .com/article.cfm?id=why-laughter-may-be-the-best-pain-medicine. Accessed September 14, 2012.

2. Daniel F. Kripke, "Hypnotics' Association with Mortality or Cancer: A Matched Cohort Study" 2, no. 1 (February 27, 2012). Also available at www.ncbi.nlm.nih.gov/pmc/articles/PMC3293137. Accessed October 1, 2012.

**CHAPTER 11. THE REST OF THE STORY**

1. Caldwell B. Esselstyn Jr., MD, *Prevent and Reverse Heart Disease* (New York: Avery, 2008), 4–5.

2. Jane Higdon, PhD, "Isothiocyanates," *Linus Pauling Institute Newsletter* (September 2005). Also available at http://lpi.oregonstate.edu/infocenter /phytochemicals/isothio. Accessed October 2, 2012.

3. Tambi Jarmi, MD, and Anupam Anarwal, MD, "Heme Oxygenase and Renal Disease" *Current Hypertension Reports* 11, no. 1 (2009): 56–62.

4. Joel Fuhrman, MD, *Super Immunity: The Essential Nutrition Guide for Boosting Your Body's Defenses to Live Longer, Stronger, and Disease Free* (New York: HarperOne, 2011), and Julieanna Hever, MS, RD, CPT, *The Complete Idiot's Guide to Plant-Based Nutrition* (New York: Penguin, 2011).

5. Soram Khalsa, MD, *The Vitamin D Revolution: How the Power of This Amazing Vitamin Can Change Your Life* (New York: Hay House, 2009), xi.

6. T. Colin Campbell, PhD, and Thomas M. Campbell II, *The China Study: The Most Comprehensive Study of Nutrition Ever Conducted and the Startling Implications for Diet, Weight Loss, and Long-Term Health* (Dallas, TX: BenBella, 2006).

7. Campbell and Campbell, *The China Study,* 94.

8. Campbell and Campbell, *The China Study,* 17.

# About the Author

Dr. James L. Marcum is a board-certified behavioral cardiologist with a thriving practice at the prestigious Chattanooga Heart Institute. *USA Today's* Qforma database named him one of the nation's most influential physicians. He and Charles Mills cohost *Heartwise*, a call-in radio program that airs on more than four hundred radio stations around the globe. In addition to hosting the *Ultimate Prescription* and *Heart of Health* television programs, Dr. Marcum is an in-demand speaker who specializes in boldly treading on topics normally overlooked in the highly marketed and profitable field of health care. Married with two children, Dr. Marcum lives in Chattanooga, Tennessee, and enjoys music, sports, and outdoor activities.

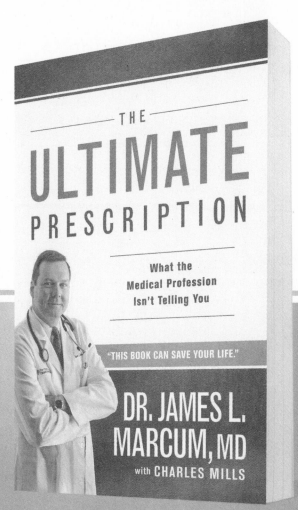

# HEARTWISE
## MINISTRIES

TRUTH | LOVE | HEALING

To continue learning visit
www.heartwiseministries.org

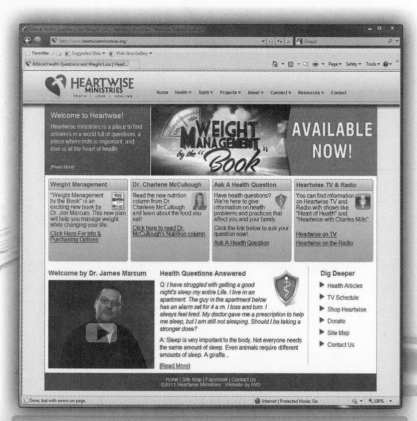